£12-95

Gudrun Paul/Birgit Hausbei/Eva-Maria Hohmann/
Michael Kahl/Claus Vögele

Aerobic Training

Meyer & Meyer Sport

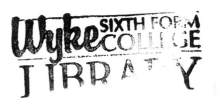

Original title: Aerobic-Training
– Aachen : Meyer und Meyer Verlag, 1998
Translated by Jean Wanko

British Library Cataloguing in Publication Data
A catalogue record for this book is available from the British Library

Paul, Gudrun ...:
Aerobic Training / Gudrun Paul and others.
– Oxford : Meyer und Meyer Sport (UK) Ltd., 2000
ISBN 1-84126-021-5

© 2000 by Meyer & Meyer Sport (UK) Ltd
Oxford, Aachen, Olten (CH), Vienna, Québec, Lansing/Michigan, Adelaide,
Auckland, Johannesburg, Budapest
Photos: Volker Minkus, Isernhagen
Graphics: Grafik-Partner, Werbung und Computer-Vertriebs GmbH,
Weiterstadt-Gräfenhausen
Cover Design: Birgit Engelen, Stolberg
Scans, Cover and Type exposure: frw, Reiner Wahlen, Aachen
Editorial: Dr. Irmgard Jaeger, Aachen, John Coghlan
Typesetting: Stone
Printed and bound in Germany
by Burg Verlag, Gastinger GmbH, Stolberg
ISBN 1-84126-021-5
e-mail: verlag@meyer-meyer-sports.com

Table of Contents

Foreword

Aerobics has established itself as one of the attractive physical activities offered in clubs, sport and fitness studios and is currently in greater demand than ever before.

One of the reasons for this is that some of the most up-to-date sports science knowledge has infiltrated the organisation of aerobics. Consequently, practical training programmes are safer and more health-promoting and thus justify their position as a viable preventative health-promoting activity.

In order to put this claim into practice, one first needs well-trained aerobics trainers; and so, bearing this in mind, an experienced teaching team of the German Gymnasts' Association has collected experience from innumerable aerobic training courses and put it into this book.

The contents comprise basic knowledge for further trainers as well as for active exercise leaders and aerobic trainers, in order to teach aerobics competently. Thus, this book is intended as a guide and source of advice, not only during a phase of intense training, but also during long-term practice in clubs, schools and studios.

Last but not least, the team of authors would like to make a wider public aware of the fascination of this kind of "sport".

Authors:
Birgit Hausbei, Eva-Maria Hohmann, Michael Kahl, Dr. Gudrun Paul, Dr. Claus Vögele.

We have chosen the female mode of address in this book, as it is mainly female trainers who are currently involved. We hope our male readers will understand.

.

1 Aerobics Today

During the course of almost two decades of constant development in aerobics, the image of this kind of activity and what it involves has noticeably developed and differentiated still further. Whereas, at the beginning of its development, aerobics was called *"whole-body fitness training"*, further development has been detected in recent years, i.e. *"aerobics as competitive sport"*. Both types of development have a lot in common, but differ in a number of significant aspects.

A third use of aerobics, especially more and more popular in North and South America, is to use aerobics as a technical foundation for specific kinds of sport such as tennis, soccer etc. By using a certain pattern of training suited to these particular sports, aerobics can also become part of the training programme of competitive sportmen. As this area of application is rare in Europe so far, we will confine ourselves to just mentioning it.

1.1 Aerobics as Whole-body Fitness Training

Reaching today's level of recognition and development was not always easy. When we look back, we can see that the level of training developed at the end of the 1970's produced a previously unknown kind of movement in the industrialised countries, as much through its being a novelty (gymnastic movements and music contained into an endurance-orientated training programme) as well as by successful marketing concepts.

Several factors like insufficient knowledge on the part of the exercise leaders and aerobic trainers, too much stress, insufficient stress differentiation in groups which were often too big etc. led to aerobic programmes often being criticised for health reasons. After aerobics seemed to have died a natural death at least in Germany at the start of the 1980's, the realisation and intensification of, and qualification for, training led to an unexpected renaissance.

Aerobics became what it is today i.e. a preventative, health-promoting kind of fitness training, which gives pleasure, fun and a sense of well-being to all kinds of participating target groups. Or, put in a different way:

"Aerobics is an effective way of training the whole body, where endurance training is at the centre, and intrinsic fitness components like strength, flexibility and co-ordination are closely combined with music in a training programme which is put together logically."

At present, aerobic programmes on offer in clubs sport and fitness studios a wide spectrum. A variety of terms describe the various mobility programmes. An attempt at structuring makes clear the following:

1. It becomes increasingly necessary to differentiate between groups of beginners and the more advanced, which is to be recommended for reasons of individual training structure and for health reasons.

2. Sometimes one detects a more pronounced use of dance forms, and sometimes the emphasis is on more athletic exercises, with and without additional apparatus. There are no great deviations in the intended sport-physiological effects here, but rather more differences are to be found in the methodical construction of training programmes, the use of newly-developed apparatus, like step, slide, the type of movements and movement techniques.

In the following section some of these trends will be introduced briefly, without claiming to be a comprehensive survey.

Alongside the *"classic aerobics lessons"* which are obviously at the heart of any basic training, the following work out forms are enjoying increased popularity.

Dance Aerobics

Funk aerobics, city jam, hip hop, cardio-funk, Latin-aerobics, Afro-aerobics, Samba-aerobics etc, are examples of dance variations in aerobic sport.

What characterises such lessons is the relationship between dance forms of movement and styles in connection with the appropiate music. A sort of choreographic programme often emerges at the end of such a session.

During these dance variations, the types of movement often deviate from the classic forms of movement. Typical arm and foot techniques as well as kinds of step and body posture are used in a modified fashion and put great demands on co-ordination and body control. The music itself during these programmes has a particular fascination and motivating force for the participants.

Bringing these "dance variations" and their typical creativity into the exercise lessons ensures fun, a good atmosphere and communication within the groups.

Aerobic Programmes Emphasizing Improved Muscle Strengthering

Body-shaping, body-styling, stomach-legs-bottom programmes, body-conditioning, pump, power dumb-bell etc are all synonyms or exercise lessons which aim to improve lasting muscle power and compensate muscular disbalance. One works predominantly with one's own body weight or with easily-available extra apparatus, like rubber bands, physio bands, physio tapes, heavy hands, exertubes, body bars, long dumb-bell etc. It is vital to warm up carefully and to choose the right exercise, all within your level of competence so far (avoid counter-productive exercises).

Interval Aerobics

This aerobic kind of game represents a combination of phases of heart and circulation training (high/ low-impact aerobic) with phases of strengthening certain muscle groups. Such a training structure is seen to be very effective by experienced exercise leaders and trainers, but it does demand sufficient experience on the part of the participants.

Circuit-aerobic Programmes

Circuit-training likewise is a combination of specific strength and endurance training. At various stages, certain chosen exercises are carried out for muscle strengthening within a certain time and observing methodical principles.

Step-Aerobics

Step-aerobics is an aerobics programme which achieves intense heart and circulation training by stepping on and off a small platform (step). Step-aerobics is characterised by the powerfully athletic kind of movement, which particularly suits our male participants.

Variations like using additional apparatus (exertubes), facilitate lasting strength type of movements. Step can also be incorporated to supplement certain floor-work exercises.

Correct technique is highly important. Understanding this, alongside a safe training structure, justifies one's claim to independent training, in order to teach step-by-step aerobics to others.

Slide

This specifically athletic activity presupposes the availability of a special "sliding- mat" and sliding shoes or socks (currently in use as a type of synthetic over-shoe).
The "*sliding mat*" or sliding board is about 160 cm long and about 50 cm wide. The participants slide on this in patterns of movement resembling fast ice-skating.
As well as training heart and circulation, the muscles in leg, hip and seat areas are worked at.

Aqua-aerobics

This mobility programme in water can be categorised as "gentle" training.
Due to the resistance from the water, movements are carried out slowly, which means that the stress intensity is lower than with some of the other afore-mentioned exercises. Therefore this programme is especially suited to target groups with joint problems e.g. the overweight.

Aerobics with Elements of Combat Sports

Boxing aerobics and karate-aerobics (Kara-T-Robics) are mobility programmes in which elements and mobility structures from individual combat sports can be combined with mobility patterns from aerobics.
And so, for example, boxing aerobics is an intensive aerobics workout with boxing and kick elements, which aim for heart and circulation, muscle strength, muscle strength endurance and co-ordination training respectively. In addition, by using some sporting equipment, like boxing gloves, skipping ropes or sandbags, boxing or kick-boxing can be simulated.

The variations described here as examples clarify the variety and range of development of aerobic "sport". Some trends only last for a short time and disappear again just as quickly as they have arrived. Longer-lasting concepts will only happen if the efficacy of the training programme, the health value, a competent presentation, and the needs of people promoting the ideas, become one complete circuit.

1.2 Aerobics as a Competitive Sport

When aerobic sport was established as a fitness sport, needs were quickly aroused amongst younger people to further this kind of sport competitively.

The first competitions were held in the U.S.A. and this inspired innumerable other countries.

The German Gymnasts' Association reacted to the existing demands of the clubs and incorporated this competitive form into its popular sports programme.

Using the heading *"team-aerobics"*, the German Gymnasts' Association set up cup competitions and German Championships.

Consequently, competitive aerobics is the German Gymnasts' Association offer to individual beginners, pairs and teams (of varying ability levels), who want to pursue aerobics competitively.

The competitive exercise programme contains certain types of movement specifically for aerobics, gymnastic exercises, dance steps as well as types of athletic exercise, and particular compulsory requirements. These types of movement are set to music.

The transposition of these demands calls for a high level of endurance (heart and circulation, muscular endurance) from competitors, as well as strength skills, flexibility and co-ordinative ability, and it all requires specific training.

Certain assessment rules apply to competitions, which allow for and regulate basic demands and developments as they occur. In these assessment rules the criteria by which the judges judge the outcome of the competition are clarified.

To be successful at competitive aerobics one must have good basic knowledge of aerobic sport as described in the following chapters.

It is important to understand further concepts, like specific preparation for competitive performance, planning for training and competitions etc.

This is becoming increasingly important, as tendencies towards competitive sport are now appearing after the absorption of aerobic competitive sport into the international competition calender of the International Gymnasts' Association.

The first World Championships of this Association in competitive aerobics took place in December 1995 in Paris.

This contest has, and will also in the future, set new standards for the continuing development of this kind of sport into the future.

2 The Healthy Consequences of Aerobics

Were you to ask any of your course participants or club members why they do sport, you would probably hear a wide variety of reasons:

"Sport helps me keep my weight down."
"I'm happier with myself when I'm in good shape and my partner appreciates that as well."
"I feel more attractive, when doing sport."
"Sport relaxes me."
"One is more successful at work when in good condition."
"Doing sport regularly increases your life expectancy, because your heart is stronger."

All of these answers describe some of the psycho-social and physical consequences of sporting activity and are mainly true.

2.1 The Psycho-social Effects

Although the experts are not yet agreed on the processes involved, it has however been established that regular sport (and in particular aerobic sport), goes hand in hand with increased physical well-being. Three aspects especially have been confirmed by scientific investigations. Firstly, regular sport reduces anxiety; endurance training even has a positive effect on depressive moods. Secondly, one's work capacity and one's enjoyment of work increases. This improvement in one's feeling of self-confidence comes about because people who do regular sport, are better able to control their weight, maintain an attractive appearance and thus participate successfully in other physical activities. All of this ensures that sportively active people have a better self-image and enjoy more social advantages e.g. find it easier to make contact with people, which is all part of one's improved fitness. We would however note the following restriction: the improvement of one's psychological well-being is not directly connected to increased aerobic fitness. In more recent studies we can see predicted that an improvement in one's absorption of oxygen is directly related to the intensity of training i.e. people who go in for intensive training, achieved a greater increase their endurance capacity than people who do not train much. However, a continuous improvement in psychological well-being could be observed in people who only trained at a moderate level. These results show that improved psychological well-being is not directly related to changes in one's endurance capacity (ability to absorb oxygen). Factors, like self-confidence and a positive feeling of self-control probably also play a part in improved psychological well-being, which process is probably hindered if aerobic training is too exhausting.

The *American National Institute of Mental Health* assesses the effects of sporting activity on one's psychological health as follows:

Aerobic training
- reduces feelings of anxiety and nervousness.
- improves one's psychological condition when feeling depressed.
- is a valuable additional form of treatment during professional therapy for the severely depressed.
- reduces stress.
- improves the psychological well-being of all age-groups.

2.2 The Physiological Effects

Endurance training has a wide variety of physiological reactions, one of which is particularly interesting: sport seems to increase the body's own production of endorphine (substances similar to morphium). The results of several studies show that the euphoria, which many high-achieving sportsmen experience after intensive training, can be traced back to increased amounts of endorphine. So far it has not been proved whether this phenomenon also occurs during less-intensive training as within the framework of leisure sporting activities.

Physical exercise is likewise a significant factor in weight control. One's metabolic rate is increased by aerobic sports, as the body uses up more calories. The main use of sporting activity during the first two months of a weight reduction programme is to ensure that mainly fat and not muscular tissue is reduced. During the following months a combination of endurance training and diet leads to greater weight reduction than just dieting on its own. At the end of a weight reduction programme those who are sportively active are in a better position to realise their ideal weight than those who only diet.

Sporting activity improves one's physical condition at all ages. When older, people can normally detect an increased decline in physical ability. This reduction of endurance, strength and flexibility is partly due to the lower level of sporting activity in older people. In a long-term study in America of endurance sportsmen, carried out over several years, changes in one's physical achievement potential were investigated and compared with similar results of non-sportsmen. All participants were 50 at the start of the survey. After 18 years the sportsmens' achievement potential had hardly changed, whilst in a comparable group of non-sportsmen, there was a 1-2% loss per year of strength, endurance and flexibility. Similarly, the otherwise inevitable increase in body fat tissue and blood pressure at rest were not to be found in the sportsmens' group. These results prove that endurance training slows down the inevitable loss of physical fitness in old age.

The physical value of endurance sport carried out regularly does not only yield improved achievement potential, but a better state of health. The main value of sporting activity is in its prevention of heart and circulation disease. In innumerable studies it has already been proved that people who regularly do some kind of endurance sport suffer less often from coronary heart disease than non-sportsmen. The illness-preventing reason for this is that endurance sport has a blood pressure reducing effect, because high blood pressure is an important risk factor for a heart attack. Other ways in which sport prevents heart and circulation problems are the favourable influence on arteriosclerosis processes, or the reduction of irregular heart rhythms.

Over and above all this, sport plays an important part in overcoming day-to-day stress. Acute and chronic stress factors in everyday living lead to physical reactions to stress, which are less apparent in sportsmen than in non-sportsmen. We can confirm this from a variety of scientific investigations at the universities of Marburg and London. Reducing stress reactions is much more obvious after a long-term training programme than if one only trains irregularly for short periods of time.

The conclusions drawn about the value and relevance of endurance sport on one's health are now quite clear: regular endurance training has a positive effect on body and spirit. Beginners should undergo a medical check-up if at all possible before doing any aerobics training programme in order to clarify any risk factors. Aerobics should only be done in safe surroundings i.e. on a dry floor, and at a moderate temperature. Beginners particularly should not overexert themselves.

3 Medical Foundations

3.1 Anatomy and Physiology

3.1.1 The Supporting and Movement Structure

In a human being, bones are part of the supporting tissues which, together with bits of cartilage, make up the skeleton. The skeleton, in turn, constitutes the passive mobility structure.

Composition of a bone:

Bones are covered with a tissue-connecting bone skin (periosteum), within which are nerves and blood vessels, taking them in many minute pipes to the centre of the bone. A bone itself consists of a compact layer (bark layer) and a spongy substance (spongy bone). These indicate an architectually well-ordered construction, well-suited to the pulling and pushing forces to which a bone is subjected in its static state and from the pulling muscles.

The basic bone substance consists of mineral salts like calcium and phosphorus (inorganic), which give the bone its hardness, whilst the connecting tissues (collagenous fibres) give it its high level of durability against pulling forces.

Digression: Osteoporosis (bone decay)
Osteoporosis is a bone disease which can affect the whole skeleton, where a reduction of the bone mass takes place, as well as a deterioration in the micro-architecture of the bone fabric. This leads to a brittleness of the bones, which again leads to greater

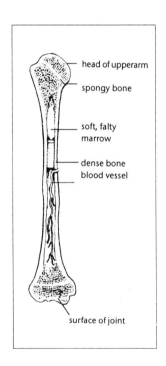

head of upperarm

spongy bone

soft, falty marrow

dense bone blood vessel

surface of joint

Diagram 1: Sketch of a tubular bone "upperarm bone" in longitudinal section

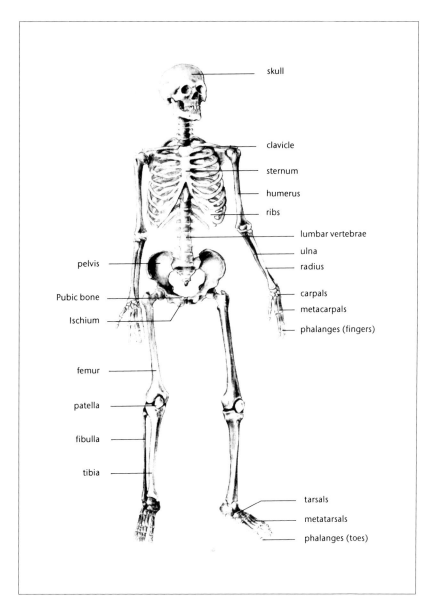

Diagram 2: Drawing of a "bone man" with labels

risk of fracture. Osteoporosis frequently afflicts women after the menopause, where one of the causes is a loss of oestrogen (reduced ovary function). These hormones are vital for the storing of minerals, especially calcium in the bones. Due to the shortage of minerals, a negative balance arises between bone creation and bone resorption.

Skeleton

Depending on their shape, one distinguishes between:
1. Tube bones or long bones (e.g. femur and humerus).
2. Flat or wide bones (e.g. skull, pelvic bone and scapula (shoulder blades).
3. Short bones (e.g. hand and foot bones).

Joints

The correct term for joining bones together is joints (diarthrosis).
   A joint consists of:
1. The surface area of the bones, which are covered in cartilage to reduce the joint areas rubbing together.
2. The joint capsule, a skin of connecting tissue, which separates the joint from the outside. This joint has two layers, an inner one (synovial membrane) which separates off the synovial fluid (this nourishes the cartilage) and the outer layer of fibre (fibrous membrane).
3. The join ligaments, which inhibit certain movements and are stored up in the capsule.

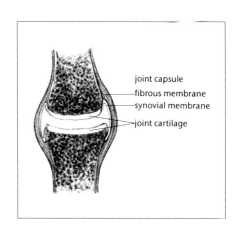

joint capsule
fibrous membrane
synovial membrane
joint cartilage

Diagram 3: Drawing of a joint and its construction with labels

Types of Joint

1. Ball-and-socket joint

Ball-and-socket joints have three axes which allow six main movements: extension, flexion, adduction and abduction, movements in- and outwards. Examples are the hip and shoulder joints.

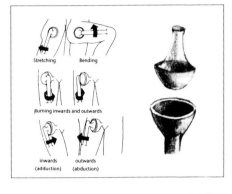

2. Socket joint

Socket joints have two axes and four main movements are possible: extension, flexion, adduction and abduction: examples are the wrist and both joints between atlas (neck vertebrae) and condylus lateralis (back of neck).

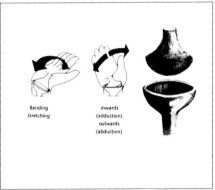

3. Hinge joint

Hinge joints have an axis making two movements possible (extension and flexion). Examples are the elbow joint, the knee joint, the upper ankle joint, and the finger joints.

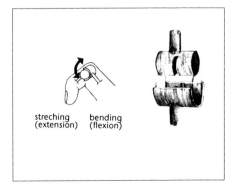

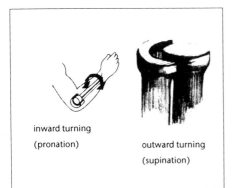

inward turning
(pronation)

outward turning
(supination)

4. Pivot or pin joint
Pivot joints have an axis which makes outward and inward turning possible (supination and pronation). Examples are in the lower arm (ulna against radius), and the first and second neck vertebrae (atlas and axis).

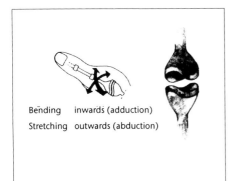

Bending   inwards (adduction)
Stretching   outwards (abduction)

5. Saddle joints
Saddle joints have two axes, making two movements on two different planes possible (extension and flexion, adduction and abduction). An example is the basic thumb joint.

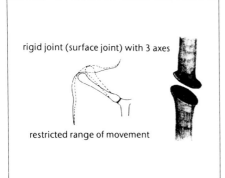

rigid joint (surface joint) with 3 axes

restricted range of movement

6. Rigid joint (surface joint)
Rigid joints present a special kind of joint. They have flat surface areas and a restricted range of movement due to their strong and taut system of ligaments. Examples are the sacrum, ilium, and the bone connections between hand and foot carpals.

Ligaments

Ligaments are predominantly found around joints and there are three different types i.e. from their mechanism point of view:

1. Strengthening ligaments (strengthen the joint capsule).
2. Leading ligaments (determine the type and extent of joint movement).
3. Restricting ligaments (restrict the extent of joint movement).

Ligaments consist of tug-resistant bundles of tissue. When they lose their elasticity, there is a greater risk of rupture (e.g. outer ankle ligaments).

Spinal Column

The spinal column constitutes the body's movable axis, carrying the head and the ribs, and containing the spinal fluid protected within the spinal canal. Its double S formation and the elasticity of the intervertebral discs are well able to cope with knocks and bumps. The spinal column consists of 24 vertebrae:
Seven neck vertebrae (lordoris), twelve chest vertebrae (kyphosis) and five pelvic vertebrae (lordosis).

The vertebrae of the sternum coccyx (kyphosis) are fused together. The vertebral column only becomes movable by means of little vertebral joints, which connect the vertebrae together. It is between the

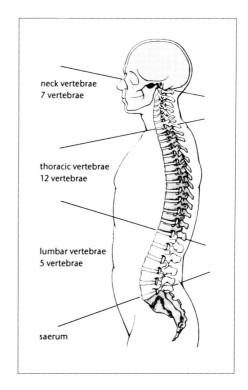

neck vertebrae
7 vertebrae

thoracic vertebrae
12 vertebrae

lumbar vertebrae
5 vertebrae

saerum

Diagram 10: Spinal column profile

skull and atlas (first neck vertebra) that nodding movements take place, and between the atlas and axis (second neck vertebra) that the head's turning movements occur. The mobility of the neck vertebrae is the greatest, but it is here that wear and tear happens fastest. The chest vertebrae permit turning movements and the lumbar area permits forward, backward and sideways movements.

Construction of a Vertebra

1. Vertebra (corpus vertebrae – where the inter-vertebral discs are attached).
2. Centrum (arcus vertebrae).
3. Dorsal process (processus spinosus).
4. Two transverse processes (processus transversi).
5. Two lower surfaces for articulation with next vertebra (processus articulares).
6. Spinal canal (canalis vertebralis – where the spinal cord runs through).

The transverse processes of the chest vertebrae carry the joint areas for the ribs to be attached.

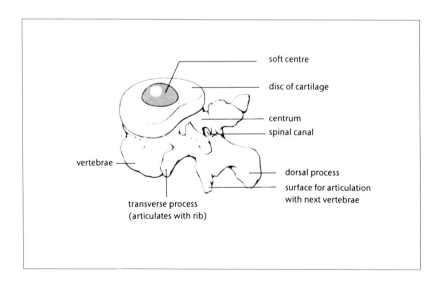

Diagram 11: Vertebrae with inter-vertebral disc

The Inter-vertebral Disc

1. Fibre-rich cartilage tissue (anulus fibrosus).
2. Soft, gelatinous centre (nucleus pulposus).

This centre is resistant to jolting due to its elasticity, and strengthens the mobility of the spinal column. As one gets older this centre loses its elasticity and contains less fluid.

Due to the taut ligaments between two vertebrae mobility is relatively slight but, in collaboration with lots of individual movements, the spinal column is very flexible.

    Throughout its length, at the back and at the front, the spinal column is encased in tight ligaments to increase its firmness.

The most Frequent Curvatures of the Spine

Hyperkyphosis: strong curvature of the thoracic vertebrae backwards (humpback).

Hyperlordosis: strong curvature of the spinal column forwards, frequently in the lumbar region (hollow back).

Scoliosis: curvature of the thoracic vertebrae to the side, usually with torsion or turning of individual vertebrae.

Digression: disease of the inter-vertebral discs
The normal wear and tear of these discs due to aging can be accelerated by incorrect body stress (e.g. wrong posture, sitting for hours on end and lack of movement). This often results in damage to the inter-vertebral discs.

One distinguishes between:

1. Prolapse, where the ring of cartilage tears and the gelatinous centre comes out backwards or sideways.
2. Protusion, where the outer ring of cartilage remains intact, but part of the disc arches forwards. Due to pressure on the exposed nerve roots, the natural consequence is pain and increased sensitivity, as well as loss of muscle power in the affected parts of the body.

3.1.2 Basic Planes, Axes and Directions of Movement

1. Frontal plane
2. Sagital plane
   (arrow direction)
3. Transverse plane

Directions of movement and their specialist terms:

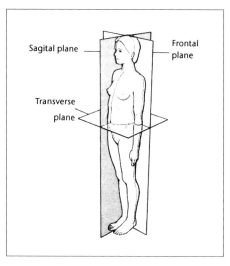

Flexion – bending a joint
Extension – stretching a joint
Abduction – sideways lifting of the extremities (arms and legs)
Adduction – pulling in the extremities
Anteversion – lifting forwards e.g. an arm
Retroversion – lifting backwards e.g. an arm
Rotation – turning

Diagram 12: Human with the different planes

Torsion – twisting
Supination – turning outwards (foot/hand e.g. palm of hand facing upwards)
Pronation – turning inwards (foot/hand e.g. back of hand facing upwards)
Dorsal flexion – bending the upper ankle
Plantar flexion – stretching the upper ankle
Lateral flexion – bending the trunk sideways
Ventral flexion – bending the trunk forwards.

3.1.3 Muscles

The muscles belong to the active mobility apparatus where the skeletal muscles constitute the main part of the human muscle structure.

They run in crossways strips, made up of innumerable individual muscles, whose job it is to effect movements in part of the bone structure, and to guarantee certain body positions during movement or when at rest.

Other muscles are the smooth muscles (inner organs and vessels and the heart muscles).

Structure of the Skeletal Muscles

There is a cover of connecting tissue round the skeletal muscles (muscle facia – perimysium externum), whose job is to give the muscle its shape.

If you cut open a muscle you can see that it is composed of bundles of fibre (myone) which are also covered in a layer of connecting tissue (perimysium internum). You can only see these muscle fibres under a microscope and they are surrounded by a thin skin of elastic fibres (endomysim). These muscle fibres are called muscle cells, which consist of so-called myofibrilli (little fibres), which in their turn consist of evenly-arranged myofilaments (even smaller than fibrilli). There are two kinds of filaments: actin (thinner and transparent) and myosin (thicker and darker). These lend the muscles their crossways-striped appearance.

If a muscle contracts, the actin filaments in between the myosin filaments are pulled, resulting in a contraction and thickening of the muscle.

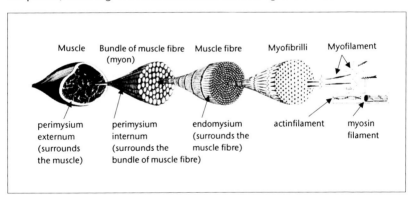

Diagram 13: Structure of a muscle

Types of Muscle Fibre

The human muscle comprises various muscle fibres, which are categorised according to their speed of contraction and resistence to tiredness.

Muscle-fibre type 1 (Slow Twitch – ST fibres)
This type of fibre is rich in myoglobin and is therefore red (oxygen-binding). Due to its many mitochondria (the body's power stations) it is responsible for

the aerob provision of energy. The ST fibres contract slowly and are capable of long-term work

Muscle-fibre type 2 (Fast Twitch - FT fibres)
This sort of fibres is poor in myoglobin and is white, has less mitochondria than type I and therefore works anaerobically. The FT fibres can contract quickly and are not capable of long-term work.

This type of fibres can be subdivided into the categories: Type 2a, 2b and 2c = intermediary fibres. Fibre types 1 and 2 are always present in the skeletal muscles, although more type 2 muscles are found in the extremities and more type 1 muscles in the trunk.

It has been proved that muscle fibres type 2 predominate in maximum and power sportsmen, whereas type 1 is to be found in endurance sportsmen. One can conclude that shifting of available muscle fibres is possible by appropriate training.

Tendons

The muscles do not usually join onto the bones, but carry on beyond the end of the bones into the tendons, which usually join onto the periosteum or the joint capsules. The tendons transmit the pulling effect of the muscle to the bones. Tendons are thinner than their own muscles and extraordinarily tensile. Tendons consist of collagenous fibres without many blood vessels. Compared with muscles they cannot be stretched as far.

Tendons based on bones are regularly surrounded by tendon sheaths (vagina tendinum) e.g. the finger and toe muscle tendons. So that tendons do not chafe and can glide well in the tendon sheath, they are surrounded by synovial fluid.

A fluid bag (bursa synovialis) provides further protection for the tendons. These are little sacks of varying sizes full of synovial fluid and with the function of a water cushion. Otherwise, the constant pressure of tendon on bone would cause the bone to disintegrate at the affected point. The tendon, on the other hand is often protected by an elastic piece of cartilage on the side facing the bone. During training one can increase the firmness of the tissue by stress adaption and thus a hypertrophy (or "feeding") of the tissue. The state of hypertrophy thus attained is less than that of the muscle. If one applies too much mechanical stress, this can cause inflammation of the sliding mechanism and greatly inhibit movements in this area e.g. inflammation of the Achilles' tendon.

Types of Muscle Power

One can distinguish between two types of muscle work: static and dynamic.

Static (Isometric) Muscle Training
Here there is no obvious muscle contraction. The length of muscle does not alter, but a high level of tension develops in the muscle. During isometric training one acquires a fast increase in strength, but muscle co-ordination is not trained. If the static muscle power is stressed from 15% to 50%, then the circulation of blood through the muscle is impaired and local acquisition of energy varies from aerobic to anaerobic. The higher the muscle tension the greater the obstruction in the vessels and thus energy is acquired anaerobically.

Example: the hands are pressed together as hard as possible out in front of the body and held there for a while.

Dynamic (Isotonic) Muscle Contraction
Here we have obvious contraction. The length of muscle changes, but the muscle tension remains the same.

One differentiates between two kinds of dynamic muscle training:
1. Positive dynamic strength: concentric or overcoming strength. The muscle contracts e.g. climbing up the horizontal bars or lifting a weight during biceps curl.
2. Negative dynamic strength: excentric or yielding strength. The muscle lengthens during similar muscle tension e.g. slowly coming down horizontal bars or letting a weight come down during biceps curl.

An advantage of this sort of muscle work is for training muscle co-ordination. Local dynamic muscle endurance is the motoric form of stress which can be trained hardest. Its starting position in untrained people can be improved by several thousand percent.

The muscle which contracts and does the most work is the agonist. Its opponent, responsible for the opposing movement, is called the antagonist. Muscles similarly involved in carrying out the movement are known as synergists (collaborators).

Main Muscle Groups and Their Functions

A. Trunk muscles
The chest muscles, stomach muscles, back muscles, neck and head muscles belong to this group.
B. Muscles of the upper and lower extremities
The leg and arm muscles belong to this group.

- M. trapezius (hooded muscle): pulls the shoulder-blade up, back and down.
- M. rhomboideus (rhombic muscle): pulls the shoulder-blade towards the spinal column.
- M. latissimus dorsi (wide back muscle): rotation inwards, adduction and retroversion of the arm.
- M. erector spinae (back stretcher): stretches the back and keeps it straight.
- M. pectoralis major: (large thoracic muscle): arm adduction in the transverse plane and rotation inwards.
- M. serratus anterior (sideways sawing muscle): pulls the shoulder-blade forwards and turns the bottom corner of the shoulder-blade outwards.
- M. rectus abdominis (straight stomach muscle): brings the rib-cage towards the pelvis.
- M. obliquus externus and internus (diagonal inner and outer stomach muscle): sideways moving and turning of the trunk.
- M. transversus abdominis (crossways stomach muscle): is also responsible for pressing the stomach organs together.
- M. iliopsoas (pelvic and hip muscle): flexion in the hip joint.
- M. gluteus maximus (large bottom muscle): hip extension, outward rotation of leg.
- Abductor group – m. gluteus medius (middle bottom muscle), m. gluteus minimus (small bottom muscle), m. tensor fasciae latae (stretcher of the high ligature): abduction, rotation outwards and inwards of the leg.

Diagram 14: Muscle man from the front and behind

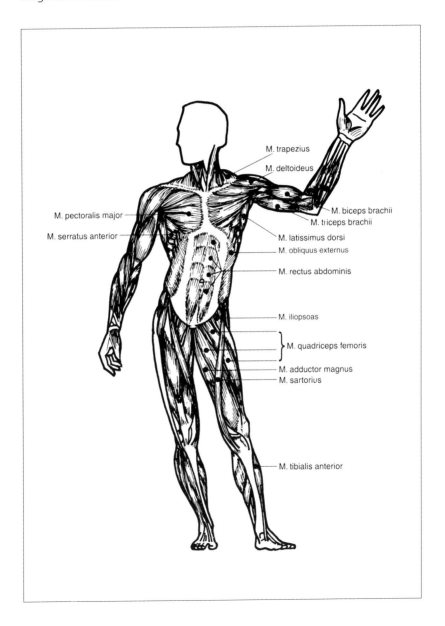

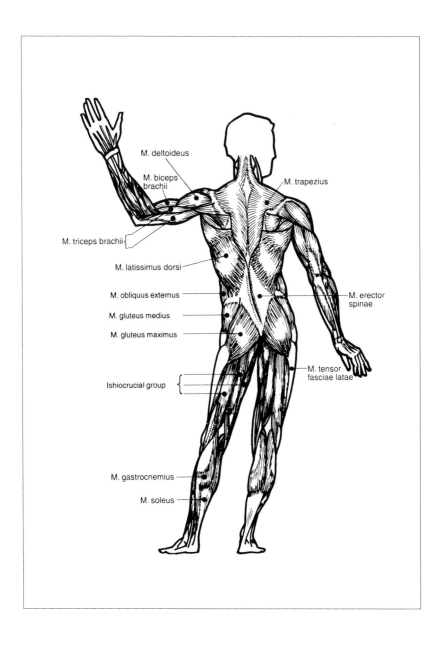

- Adductor group – m. adductor longus (long thigh puller), m. adductor brevis (short thigh puller), m. adductor magnus (big thigh puller): adduction and outward rotation of the leg.
- M. quadriceps femoris (quadriceps thigh stretcher): extension of knee joint, flexion of hip joint. Its four muscles are called: m. rectus femoris, m. vastus mediales, m. vastus lateralis, m. vastus intermedius.
- M. sartorius (cutter muscle): anteversion, abduction and outward rotation of hip joint, flexion of the knee joint and inward rotation of the skin.
- Ischiocrural group – m. biceps femoris (double-headed thigh muscle), m. semitendinosus (half tendon muscle), m. semimembranosus (flat tendon muscle) – all take part in flexing and rotating outwards and inwards the bent shin, as well as extension of the hip joint.
- M. gastrocnemius (the twin calf muscle): flexing the knee joint and flexing towards the sole of the foot at the ankle joint, ends in the Achilles' tendon.
- M. soleus (layered muscle): flexing towards the sole of the foot at the ankle joint, ends in the Achilles' tendon.
- M. tibialis anterior (front shin muscle): dorsal flexion and supination of the foot.
- M. deltoideus (delta muscle): abduction, lifts the arm in all directions as far as horizontal.
- M. biceps brachii (double-headed arm muscle): flexion and supination in the lower arm, anteversion in the upper arm.
- M. triceps brachii (triple-headed arm stretcher): extension of the lower arm and retroversion of the upper arm.

3.1.4 The Heart and Circulatory System

So that all the muscles receive an adequate supply of oxygen and nourishment, and so that the blood can be brought right into all the cells, the organism needs a special kind of circulatory system.

Structure of the Circulatory System

The heart is the circulation's motor. The blood is dispersed throughout the body via the arteries. The aorta comes out of left-hand chamber of the heart (left ventricle) and supplies the body's main circulatory system with nourishment and oxygen-rich blood. The exchange of the supply of

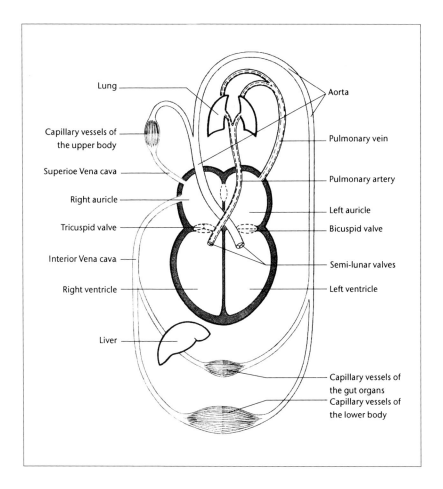

Diagram 15: Blood circulatory system

oxygen and all the nourishment takes place in the capillaries. The pulmonary artery comes out of the right-hand chamber of the heart (right ventricle) and goes to the lung, where the blood is re-supplied with oxygen from the aveoli. The blood, now rich in oxygen is taken via the pulmonary vein into the left auricle. The veins are responsible for bringing the body's blood (reduced in oxygen) back, and they do this via the inferior vena cava and on into the heart's right auricle.

The arteries are the vessels which carry the blood away from the heart to the lungs or into the peripheries. The vessels, which bring the blood to the heart (from the lungs or other organs) are called veins. The terms have nothing to do with the abundance or lack of oxygen in the blood being transported.

Oxygen (O_2) is carried by the red blood corpuscles (erythrocytes), which consist of a basic substance, protein-rich and the red-coloured matter, haemoglobin, to which the oxygen adheres.

Structure and Function of the Heart

The heart is a muscular hollow organ which represents a suction and pressure pump. It regulates with certain valves the blood's direction of flow. Two-thirds of the heart are in the left-hand side of chest and one third on the right. The vertical axis runs from top back right to bottom front left. It is approximately the same size as the clenched fist of its owner and is about 300 grams in weight. It is divided into two halves by a connecting wall i.e. the right-hand side and left-hand side. Another crossways wall divides each half of the heart into an auricle and a ventricle. The heart valves off the auricle from the ventricle, so that the blood cannot rush back. The blood flows out of the right auricle through the right ventricle into the pulmonary artery and from the left auricle into the left ventricle to the aorta.

The wall of the heart has three layers:

- Heart interior skin (endocardium)
- Heart muscle (myocardium)
- Outer skin (epicardium)
- The heart itself lies in a heart bag (pericardium).

The heart muscle belongs to the crossways-strip muscles, but is not part of the skeletal muscle system. The contraction of the heart muscle is regulated by its own stimulus system, but the heart rate can be accelerated or slowed down by influences on the vegetative nervous system. The coronary vessels are responsible for looking after the heart's blood supply and, if these are blocked (e.g. by narrowing their width), then there is a lack of oxygen which can cause a heart attack.

The heart muscle increases its size in sportsmen i.e. the ventricles expand, the heart wall thickens and can achieve more.

Heart performance: at rest the heart transports about five litres of blood per minute, but when exercising this can be increased to between 25 and 40 litres per minute depending on the training level of the person concerned.

There are two phases of heart activity:

1. Systole (contraction of the heart), also known as driving-out phase. The blood flows from the auricles into the ventricles. During the systole of the ventricles, the blood is driven into the pulmonary aorta.
2. Diastole (expansion of the heart), also known as stretching phase. When the auricles stretch, the blood flows from the peripheries and the lungs into both auricles i.e. if the auricles contract, the ventricles stretch and vice versa.

The systolic blood pressure in the aorta is 150 mm on the mercury scale (Hg). In the peripheries, the blood pressure is measured with a blood pressure measuring device. The blood measure cuff is put around the upper arm and pumped up. When the air is let out, the systolic (upper) rate is around 110-140 mm/Hg and the diastolic (lower) rate around 70-90 mm/Hg.

If the readings are above 160 mm/Hg systolic and 90 mm diastolic, one talks about high blood pressure (hypertension), but if it is under 110 mm/Hg it is known as low blood pressure (hypotension). Hypertonie is dangerous as it can lead to a heart attack.

Blood pressure is dependent of the power of heart activity (what it "throws out") and also the peripheral resistance of the blood vessels.

The pulse matches the impulse of the blood-flow in the blood vessels, mainly in the arteries. The heart propels with each beat a certain amount of blood under pressure into the peripheries and one can then measure this pulse from the arteries.

In adults, the resting pulse is about 60-80 beats per minute, which can rise to over 100 beats per minute during physical exercise or emotional stimulation.

If one is well-trained the pulse can fall to 50 beats per minute without causing any illness, and the heart then works more economically.

3.1.5 The Lung

When one breathes in air passes down the trachea through the bronchial passages to the lung lobes.

The lung is a spongy organ which fits neatly into the chest cavity, and there are right and left lobes of the lung. The right-hand lobe has three flanges and the left-hand one has two. As already mentioned, the exchange of gases takes place in the alveoli, which are made of a very thin layer and are surrounded by a network of capillaries. When one breathes in, oxygen (O_2) is taken in and carbon dioxide is then breathed out.

The total amount of air breathed in is never used for the exchange of gases, but only the air which reaches the alveoli. Also, during breathing out all the air is not pressed out of the lungs, but quite a large amount remains behind.

An adult at rest ideally needs 6-8 litres of air per minute to be supplied with oxygen, and during physical exercise consumption rises to 120 litres per minute. Well-trained people need up to 250 litres per minute.

3.1.6 Energy Supply

The lung i.e. one 's breathing as well as one's circulation are in fact aids to ensure that one's metabolism is supplied with enough oxygen and other substances, as well as getting rid of intermediate and end products.

The muscle cell (muscle fibre) consists of fibrilli (myofibrilli) running parallel to each other, as already mentioned, which lie in the sarcoplasm (a fluid containing electrolites and proteins). This is where the anaerobic supply of energy comes from (without oxygen). Mitochondria (the cell's "power stations") and other subcellular structures can be found in the sarcoplasm. The aerobic combustion of energy-rich substances takes place in the mitochondria.

The energy one needs for the vital cell processes cannot be obtained directly from one's food, but must be turned into energy-rich phosphate compounds.

The two transporters of this are:
- Adenosintriphosphate (ATP): delivers energy directly to all the necessary energy processes.
- Creatinphosphate (CP):
  refills the empty ATP reserves by resynthetising.

The myosin molecule depends on the chemical energy of the ATP's for its mechanical work. Other energy transporters cannot be used by the body straight away and must be transformed. The first amount of energy comes from the fission of ATP. The ATP supply to the cell is of limited duration: 2-3 seconds.

The muscle fibre uses various ways of re-synthetising the ATP. ADP (adenosindiphosphate) is produced from the splitting-off of an energy-rich phosphate compound.

$$ATP + H_2O = ADP + P$$

To facilitate further muscle work, the ATP is refilled (creatinase) from the creatin-phospate-supply

$$KP + ADP \ (creatinase) = creatin + ATP$$

Overall, the energy-rich phosphates (ATP and KP) enable a maximum working time of ten seconds. If these are exhausted ATP is supplied via other energy-supply mechanisms.

One distinguishes between anaerobic energy supply (without oxygen) and aerobic supply (with oxygen).

1. Anaerobic Energy Supply
The anaerobic energy supply happens in the sarcoplasm by using glucose (carbohydrate) without oxygen and is thus known as anaerobic glycolysis. Here, only glucose i.e. glycogen (the way glucose is stored in the liver and muscle cell) can be used. Due to the anaerobic disposal of glucose, lactate appears as a waste product as a result of intense muscular activity. When the lactate level in the cell and blood rises, overacidity (acidosis) occurs, which affects the cell's metabolism. The energy supply to the cell stagnates and physical exercise ceases rapidly.

$$ATP + lactic \ acid$$

During anaerobic glycolysis only 2 mol ATP per mol glucose is produced.

2. Aerobic Energy Supply

During the aerobic supply of energy, carbohydrates (glucose) and fats (fatty acids) are burnt up: Only in extreme situations (e.g. hunger and intense long-term stress) are proteins (amino acids) also used. This process takes place in the mitochondria. During decomposition (oxidative combustion) with oxygen the following happens:

$$ATP + CO_2 \text{ (carbon dioxide)} + H_2O \text{ (water)}$$

Water is secreted and carbon dioxide breathed out. During the aerobic oxidation of glucose (aerobic glycolysis) 38 mol ATP are produced per mol glucose. In the combustion of fats, about 100 mol ATP are produced per mol fatty acid. It is obvious that the greatest energy production comes from aerobic combustion. Anaerobic glycolysis gives an even faster supply of energy.

Connection between energy supply and physical exertion:

1. Extremely Short Exertion (up to ten Seconds)

Energy supply comes from getting rid of ATP and KP reserves (the body's own reserves of energy). During this time (intense exertion) there is a high intake of oxygen, but accelerated breathing does not occur. The amount of oxygen used at this time but not absorbed, is called "oxygen debt", which remains until the work is over and is then breathed in.

2. Maximum Exertion of up to three Minutes

The energy required must now come from anaerobic glycolysis. After about 40 seconds, maximum energy supply is attained. If the intensity of work is maintained, then the lactate level in the blood rises and the stress must cease.

3. Medium Exertion of up to 20 Minutes

The energy for medium exertion is mainly covered by the aerobic oxidation of glucose (aerobic glycolyse). Absorption of oxygen and its use is now in a so-called "steady state" i.e. it is balanced out. After about 20 minutes, the combustion of fatty acids increases and so the intensity decreases.

If the intensity is subsequently increased, one's energy supply must come from anaerobic oxidation again.

4. Long-term Exertion up to an Hour:
The supply of energy comes mainly from the combustion of fatty acids. Oxygen consumption rises by about 15%. One notices less capacity for work and the intensity of exertion must be reduced, so that the glycogen reserves are preserved.

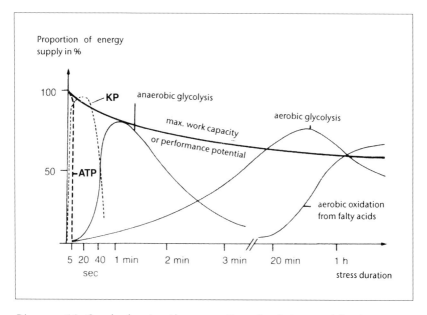

Diagram 16: Graph showing the proportion of substances delivering energy during physical exertion of varying lengths, including maximum performance potential at any one time.

In conclusion, one can see that the primary source of energy ATP is filled up in order by KP, anaerobic glycolysis and then the aerobic energy supply. Acquiring energy does not happen in strict order though, but rather from overlapping, depending on stress duration and intensity.

The aerobic energy supply via getting rid of glucose and fatty acids is best for the body. Waste products like carbon dioxide and water are secreted easily, there is overacidity through a rise in the lactate level, and so work (e.g. aerobics) can proceed.

3.1.7 Nourishment or Diet

The body needs a healthy and balanced diet to improve or maintain its performance potential. There is a huge range of available foods today and everything that the body needs is available in abundance. In spite of this, however, our civilised world depicts a number of illnesses connected with our diet. This is not due to insufficient exercise, but imbalanced and incorrect types of diet lead to damage to one's health.

It is no longer a secret that diet has a direct effect on a sportsman's performance. An aerobic trainer should be well-enough informed about diet to be able to help her course participants if they have any dietary enquiries.

Foodstuffs and their functions:

FOODSTUFF GROUP	FUNCTION
Carbohydrate	Energy-carriers
Fat	"Combustion" materials
Protein	"Building" materials
Bulk material	Non energy-carriers
Water	"Functional" materials
	Nourishment group
Vitamins	Non energy-carriers
Minerals	"Effective, protective and
Trace elements	regulating materials"

Essential nourishing products cannot be made in the body, they have to be taken in via our food. The essentials are water, eight amino acids (the smallest protein elements), 2 x non-saturated fatty acids, 13 vitamins and a number of minerals i.e. mixed and trace elements as well as bulk materials (roughage). The non-essentials are carbohydrates, the saturated fatty acids and the remaining amino acids. As a source of energy carbohydrates are nonetheless vital for our energy supply.

The proportion of energy is expressed in kilocalories (kcal).

Definition: A (kilo) calorie is the amount of warmth needed to warm up a litre of water from 14,5°C to 15,5°C.

On the 1ˢᵗ January 1978 a new unit , the joule, (KJ = Kilojoule) was introduced .

Definition: A (kilo) joule is the amount of work done when the target of strength (1Nm) is moved by a metre in the direction of the force.

The physiological combustion levels of basic foodstuffs are:

    1 g. carbohydrate = 4.1 kcal (17 kj.)
    1 g. fat   = 9.3 kcal (39 kj.)
    1 g. protein   = 4.1 kcal (17 kj)

As a comparison:

    1 g. alcohol   = 7.1 kcal (30 kj)

To convert calories into joules:

    1 kcal = 4.184 kj. i.e. 1. kj. = 0.239 kcal.

Basic Foodstuffs

1. Carbohydrates

Carbohydrates are the most important source of energy for our physical and mental performance and constitute in quality the main part of a balanced diet. About 50-60% of our daily calorific needs should be covered by carbohydrates.

Structure of carbohydrates:

a) Simple sugar (monosaccharin)

   e.g. fructose, glucose, galactose e.g. found in honey, fruits, drinks, sweets, milk.

b) Binate sugar (disaccharin)

   e.g. saccharose, maltose, lactose e.g. found in household sugar, jam, sweets, lemonade, malt beer, milk.

c) Compound sugar (oligosaccharin)

   e.g. maltotetrose = a mixture of sugar and dextrin

   e.g. sportmen's energy drinks, toast, crispbread, rusks.

d) Complex carbohydrate (poly saccharin)

   e.g. cellulose, starch e.g. found in rice, potatoes, cereals, muesli, bread, noodles, bananas, bulk elements from left-over grain products, fruit and vegetables.

The reabsorption of carbohydrates comes mainly in the form of monosaccharin and all other forms are first converted to these smallest elements i.e. split apart, before they are useful in producing energy.

Things which the body does not use immediately as a source of energy, it stores away as glycogen in the liver and muscles. When the body's blood sugar level falls it uses the liver's glycogen, and what it has stored in the muscles is used for physical and muscular work.

The transport of complex carbohydrates, whilst keeping one's fat level under control and being involved in sport is a prerequisite for a rich supply of glycogen to the muscles.

Simple carbohydrates like sugar and grape sugar allow the insulin level to rise in the blood. Insulin is a hormone which reduces blood sugar formed in the pancreas. Glucose is stored in the liver and muscles as well as in fatty tissues, and only a certain amount can be stored as glycogen. The rest is turned to fat in the liver and stored as fatty deposits in the tissues. So, sportsmen and non-sportsmen alike should see that they eat in accordance with their needs.

Carbohydrates should preferable be eaten in complex forms like whole-food products, potatoes and vegetables like fresh fruit. Starch should be the most important dietary carbohydrate depending on the amount eaten (DGE 1992).

Bulk foods (roughage) raise the feeling of fullness but cannot be broken down. They stimulate gut activity and are often rich in vitamins and minerals. They also have a positive influence on the blood sugarlevel. They ensure a need-orientated, constant supply of carbohydrates to muscle, nerve and brain cells.

2. Protein

Proteins are substances made up of amino acids (the smallest building unit of protein). Some amino acids are essential for the body and must be included in one's diet. Protein is the basic element of all cells, including muscle cells (actin and myosin). One's daily protein requirement is around 12% i.e. about 0.8 g. per kilo body weight of one's daily calorie intake.

One can differentiate between:

animal protein	– from meat, meat products, milk, milk products, fish, eggs, etc.
vegetable protein	– from cereals, potatoes, vegetables, pulses, nuts etc.

Animal proteins, with relatively high fat content i.e. cholesterol, (increases the danger of arteriosclerosis) and purine (increases uric acid and the danger of gout) should be avoided. Vegetable proteins such as fish and milk products are better (DGE 1992).

On the whole, we consume enough protein in a balanced diet to cover our protein needs during sport. Additional protein supplements in the form of powder etc. are unnecessary and usually very expensive (DGE 1992).

3. Fat
Fat consists of compounds of fatty acids and glycerine, representing the largest energy deposits in the human body. In conditions of extreme endurance stress, the body can fall back on its fat deposits when supplies of glycogen are exhausted.

A human being consists of a fat-free body mass (lean mass) and body fat, the combination of which is called body composition. The body fat (fat deposit) is about 11-20% of a man's body weight and about 15-25% of a woman's body weight, assuming they eat normally. The fat percentage of trained sportsmen can be much lower, depending on the type of sport.

In a balanced and healthy diet the proportion of fat in one's diet should be around 30%. The actual intake is around 40% and much too high, which then favours the offset of certain diseases and one's performance potential is reduced (overweight).

So, fats play an important role:

1. They transport fat-soluble vitamins.
2. Essential fatty acids (several non-saturated fatty acids e.g. linol acid) cannot be got rid of by the body itself. They are important for the formation of hormone cells and cell membrane structures.

Several non-saturated fatty acids are in seed oils like wheat germ oil, linseed oil, soya oil and other vegetable oils. Animal fats contain a lot of cholesterol (which encourages blood vessel disease). The consumption of these food products should therefore be restricted.

Protective and Regulating Materials

1. Vitamins
Vitamins are a group of effective products, vitally important for guiding and regulating metabolic processes. They cannot or can only be partly synthetised and must therefore be added to one's food. Vitamins belong to our essential basic nutritional needs and are organic materials.

As a result of their solubility, they can be divided into fat-soluble vitamins (A, D, E, and K) and water-soluble vitamins C, B_1, B_2, B_6, B_{12}, folic acid, pantothenic acid, niacine acid, biotine.

In recent years the consumption of fruit, vegetables, and vitamin-rich juices has adequately covered our vitamin intake. Even ordinary sportsmen do not need any additional vitamin products. Too high a dose of fat-soluble vitamins can lead to kidney damage, deposits in the blood vessels and other body damage.

2. Minerals and Trace Elements
Minerals and trace elements are inorganic matter which cannot be formed in the body. They regulate vital biological processes in the body and are lost by sweating, urine and faeces must be balanced via the diet.

Calcium, phosphorus, sodium, potassium, chlorine and magnesium belong to the mineral group.

Zinc, iron, manganese, copper, iodine, fluoride and selenium belong to the trace elements.

Sportsmen can suffer a loss of potassium and magnesium, possibly also iron when they sweat. The symptoms of this are tiredness, muscle cramps and drop in performance. All minerals and trace elements are present in a balanced diet.

Acute mineral deficiency e.g. in sportsmen, can be restored by fruit and fruit juices diluted with mineral water containing magnesium or sodium, in a ratio of 1:2 or 1:3. Generally sportsmen should not take mineral tablets without consulting a doctor, as this can lead to a fluctuation in the body's mineral supply, which also affects one's normal body functions.

3. Water

The body of the average adult consists of 60% water i.e. no life is possible without water. Even if the body loses 2% (1.4 litres) this causes reduced performance and if we lose as much as 15%, (three days without water) we die.

So, drinking is important, especially for sportsmen. They lose liquid and electrolytes e.g. potassium and magnesium by sweating. Coffee, Cola and sugary lemonades are unsuitable drinks as they increase one's thirst even more and contain no minerals or vitamins.

Recommended drink pattern for sportsmen:
a) Before starting any physical exercise the sportsman should have drunk enough, i.e. do not start with a liquid deficit.
b) In endurance sports lasting longer than 45 minutes one should sip small amounts (about 150 ml) in between times.
c) In the summer the drinks should not be too cold (12°C-20°C), and in winter slightly warmed i.e. room temperature.

3.2 Typical Aerobic Injuries

In recent years, aerobics has regained its popularity, but even here, just as in other kinds of physical activity, acute injuries or chronic problems can occur, especially in our lower limbs. To prevent injury the following points should be noted.

1. Shoes
   These must be suitable for aerobics with good cushioning at both the front of the foot, and in the heel area, have sufficient strengthening at the edge of the shoe (lateral movements), be a good fit, have easy and good rolling-away qualities, but be stable in the arch of the foot.
2. Floor-covering
   The floor-covering should not be too hard (a sprung-floor is ideal) so that any bumping or jolting of the joints is supported better.
3. Training intensity
   An extremely high level of stress e.g. high impact or insufficient warming-up leads to excessive strain and an increased risk of injury.
4. Overweight
   This leads to too great a load being put on joints, ligaments, tendons and muscles.

5. Technique
   The technique of the exercises to be practised should be clean and automatic. Mistakes often made are stepping too firmly, heels not touching the ground, knee position on landing is incorrect.
6. Wrong foot position
   e.g. fallen arches, splay foot or club-foot need good arch supports in the shoes, so that there is minimal strain on the tendons and ligaments.

Shin Splits

Anterior-tibia Syndrome
This muscle starts at the tibia and crosses the ankle joint to reach the middle edge of the foot, causing a dorsal flexion of the foot.

Definition: ischaemia – lack of oxygen supply to the muscles and damaging of the nerves in the anterior part of the tibia.
   Causes and symptoms: the extensor group in the anterior part of the tibia between skin and calf bone is covered in strong "fasciae". When the frequently weak muscle is overworked, it can cause rubbing and even muscle oedema. At its acute stage there is considerable pain and it is impossible to extend the toes backwards e.g. when walking on the heels.
   Initial remedy: if the symptoms are acute, put the leg up, keep it still and seek a doctor's advice.
   Prevention: note the tips given at the beginning about shoes, technique, volume of training etc.

Posterior-tibia Syndrome
This comes from the rear upper half of the tibia and fibula, crosses behind the middle ankle bone to the sole of the foot and is fixed to the middle bone of the foot. The muscle causes a plantar flexion and supination of the foot. Problems arise when rolling along the foot.
   Initial remedy and prevention: see "anterior-tibia syndrome".

Chondropathia Patellae

Definition: pain syndrome around the knee-cap e.g. cartilage damage to the patella. Causes and symptoms: mechanical overloading of the structures inserted at the patella, and very common in sportsmen who regularly work with knee bending. The problems regularly occur when going down mountains or climbing stairs, but also during longer knee-bending e.g. at the cinema. The pain can be localised to the rear of the knee joint, and pressurised pain or tension in the quadriceps muscle usually start it off.

Initial remedy: take away the pressure and rest it for a short time if the pain is acute. Maybe injections. Avoid knee-bending, especially with weights.

Prevention: correct technique for knee-bending and carrying out movements.

Meniscus Injuries

The menisci are layers of cartilage which serve as buffers between the femur and tibia.

Causes and symptoms: Damage or tearing of the meniscus by rotating the knee joint with the lower leg in a fixed position but with the knee bent. Shooting pain and blocking of the joint are typical, often followed by an inflammatory discharge in the joint.

Initial remedy: seek a doctor's advice immediately. Depending on the degree of damage, various treatments are available.

Prevention: carry out movements correctly and accurately and maintain good body control to minimise the danger of injury.

Inflammation of the Achilles' Tendon

The calf muscles end in the Achilles' tendon (tendo calcaneus), which is fixed to the heel bone (calcaneus). The muscles cause plantar flexion, supination and adduction of the foot.

Definition: pain in the distal part of the Achilles' tendon.

Causes and symptoms: the majority of problems are caused by degenerative changes in connection with a chronic reaction to overloading, too hard a floor, and poor shoes. Considerable pain can stem from acute irritation leading to an inability to walk. The foot is held in tiptoe position, thus helping the tendon to recover. The whole area is sensitive to pressure, overwarm and reddened. One complains of difficulty in walking in the morning, particularly when rolling off the foot. In chronic variations the above problems keep on occuring. The lower part of the Achilles' tendon is swollen reducing the moving about of the sliding tissue.

Initial remedy: at the acute stage it is put in plaster or strapped up with the foot in tiptoe position, as well as administering pain-killers and medicaments to reduce the swelling. Cortisone injections into the tendon are dubious due to the danger of rupture. At the chronic stage, electrotherapy and bandaging with ointment can help. One must reduce training, and then gradually increase again after symptoms have subsided.

Prevention: stretching, inlays to correct wrong foot positions, correct technique, springy floor as well as well-cushioned shoes are important.

Pulled or Strained Muscles
Causes and symptoms: insufficient warming-up before the main part of training, as well as inadequate or wrong stretching of the muscles after training, promote the risk of injury. Also, injuries can more easily occur from tiredness and the subsequent break-down of co-ordination and technical errors. With slight strains, one only senses some pulling or a feeling of tension in the muscle, but a sudden localised pain and swelling must be regarded as a more serious strain.

Initial remedy: if it is a bad strain, quieten down the respective extremity and seek a doctor's advice. With less serious problems, cease training until all pain has disappeared, then start again carefully. No massage in this area!

Prevention: see causes.

Inflammation of the Vocal Chords
Causes and symptoms: overexerting the voice due to too many courses and wrong technique. If the music is very loud, the voice must be raised considerably. Also, too much use of the voice in cueing can lead to straining it. Indications of a vocal chords problem are: a hoarse voice (also in the mornings), reduction in sonority, swallowing problems, a sore throat and speech problems. To moisten the vocal chords, the body produces more saliva, which in turn causes frequent coughing. By coughing to get rid of the soliva, the vocal chords suffer again. If these symptoms are ignored, total loss of voice can ensue.

Immediate remedy: If the person is in great pain, an ear-nose-and-throat specialist should be consulted.

Prevention: breathing and speech training from a speech therapist. If possible, use a microphone or muffle the volume of the music.

Tiredness Fracture
Definition: fractures of the bones in the foot resulting from long-term and/or non-physiological exertion.

Causes and symptoms: especially when a sudden load is put on the bones in the foot and the appropriate biological adaptation does not take place, then a so-called tiredness fracture in the metatarsal bones occurs. Restricted movement, long-lasting, localised pain with swelling and reddening of the affected area.

Immediate remedy: tiredness fractures are dealt with by putting the foot in plaster, which usually gives speedy recovery to the tiredness zones.

Prevention: start training again in stages, increasing gradually in order to secure the right biological adaptation.

Inflammation of the Tendon Sheath (Tendovaginitis)
Definition: an inflammation of the tendon sheath usually caused by irritation and overworking.

Causes and symptoms: as a result of mechanical overexertion, a water-retaining swelling of the tissues of the tendon sheath takes place and hurts whenever one moves. The secretion of fibrin (fibrus material in the blood) explains the crunching sensation in the sheath whenever one moves.

Initial remedy: rest the affected limb until the pain eases, then gradually work it again.

Prevention: balanced training, to avoid partial overloading.

Shoulder Problems (Biceps-tendon Syndrome)
Definition: collective term for painful injury in the long biceps tendon.

Causes and symptoms: The long biceps tendon runs in a narrow channel (sulcus intertubercularis) in close anatomical connection with the rotating collar (muscle group of the shoulder joint). As the channel is relatively narrow, inflammation and degenerative variations can occur e.g. caused by fast, uncontrolled movements and repetitive movements over the head. Pain occurs in the shoulder, painful pressure-point at the biceps tendon, or when tensing the biceps upwards, arm movements are restricted. There is danger of rupturing the biceps tendon if degenerative damage happens first.

Initial remedy: rest until pain stops and do not allow steroid injections into the tendon because of danger of rupture. Slow resumption of training.

Prevention: balanced training, good warming-up of the shoulder muscles.

Listen carefully to your body, taking note of the slightest pain or discomfort, and always let it heal. Reduce your volume of training until that happens. The symptoms of injury have probably been covered by a higher emission of adrenalin, so the injury damage could increase. Go to a specialist doctor if the pain lasts or reoccurs despite immediate treatment. Pay attention to correct technique and all other points mentioned at the beginning.

With acute sporting injuries, the following steps should be taken immediately:

1. Rest the affected part of the body, maybe put it up e.g. a leg.
2. Use cooling down procedures (damp, cool towels, even better an ice pack or ice cubes).
3. Maybe a compress bandage.

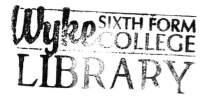

4 Some Basic Specifically-aerobic Principles

4.1 Basic Movement Pattern

4.1.1 Body Posture

Good upright body posture prevents incorrect loading of both the passive mobility structure (especially the spinal column) and the active mobility structure (muscles). It is characterised by observance of the physiological swinging of the spinal column with compensatory muscular balancing of all the muscle groups involved.

One can learn a lot about a person's personality from his posture i.e. good body posture reflects a balanced, harmonious, self-assured way of life.

If a vertical plumb-line were to be drawn through the body, good posture is indicated by two symmetric halves when seen from the front. Seen from the side, the plumb-line runs through the shoulder, hip and knee joints as well as the arches of the feet.

The typically aerobic starting position when standing is characterised as follows:

- Legs stand apart a bit further than the width of one's hips.
- Legs and feet are turned outwards slightly, with the knee joint pointing towards the toes.
- Knee joints are slightly bent.
- The trunk is stable (tummy and bottom muscles tense).
- Both sides of the pelvis are at the same level.
- The breastbone is raised.
- The shoulder-blades are pulled back and downwards.
- Both shoulders are level.
- The neck vertebrae are stretched (crown of head towards the ceiling).

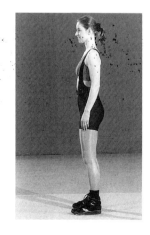

4.1.2 Technique for Doing the Movements

In order to present a credible image and fulfil the correct requirements of good teaching, every good aerobics trainer must carry out the movements clearly and precisely: the clearer the movement, the easier its execution by the participants. Mistakes and inaccuracies on the part of the trainer are then doubled by the participants.

Each movement has its precise start and finish as well as a clear mode of moving i.e. it is never tossed or "hurled" unnecessarily.

Hyperexertion (overstretching) of joints, especially knee and elbow joints and the pelvic vertebrae, are to be avoided.

During high-impact-steps (e.g. jogging) one should be especially careful to roll the feet from the ball of the foot to the heel at each contact with the ground.

Mistakes frequently occurring in carrying out step patterns are bouncing the heel of the stationary leg as well as excessive bouncing in the knee joints.

4.1.3 Basic Steps

Aerobics differentiate between low and high-impact movements. The word "impact" means "bouncing stress", So, low-impact generally means reduced stress on the joints (and spinal column), and high-impact a higher level of stress.

During low-impact at least one foot remains on the ground, but during high-impact both feet leave the ground briefly (a small flight phase).

The expressions low-impact and high-impact do not tell us anything about the intensity of training. Low-impact steps with a large range of movement and long leverage can be more intensive than high-impact movements which are kept small and supple (steering the intensity).

During the following descriptions of basic movement and step patterns, the number of necessary beats is also included.

Marching/ Walking (or March/ Walk)   *2 beats*

Marching means marching on the spot varied by opening and closing the feet (marching out-in). The high-impact version is called jogging.

   Walking implies marching on various types of path either forwards, backwards, diagonally or in a circle.

Correct performance:

- Upper body remains upright and still.
- Arms swing alternately and rhythmically at the same time.
- Knee joints remain slightly bent.
- During marching, the feet are rolled from the ball of the foot to the heel.
- When walking forwards, heels are put down first and rolled as far as the toes.
- This rolling is soft and barely audible.

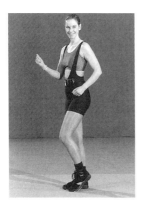 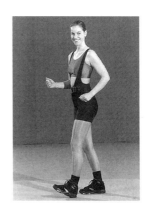

V-Step   *4 beats*

The feet trace a V-pattern on the ground. The first two steps are further apart and forwards (technique: put the heels down, feet and knees turned outwards lightly), the other two steps are much closer together backwards.

Correct performance:

- Knee joints remain slightly bent, but do not give way.

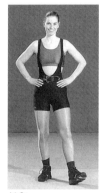 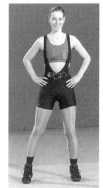 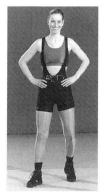 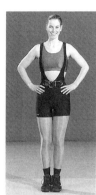

V-Step

Push Touch (or Toe Tap)   *2 beats*

One leg is placed to the side or forwards, to the back or diagonally forwards, without changing where your weight is resting; then tap the floor with the tip of your foot ("tap").

Correct performance:

- Upper body remains motionless (no change of where your weight is).
- Knee joint of the stationary leg remains slightly bent, is still and does not go on bouncing

Step Touch   *2 beats*

One leg is put out to the side (or forwards or backwards) as in Push Touch, and then one's whole body weight rests on that leg. The same leg is brought back again on the ball of the foot and rolled towards the heel. After this the other leg is drawn up and the tip of the foot taps the ground close to the stationary leg. A double sideways performance is called Double Step Touch.

Correct performance:

- Knee joints remain still and do not bounce.
- Knee joints always remain behind the tips of the feet (do not bend too far).

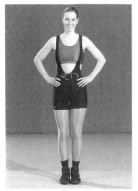 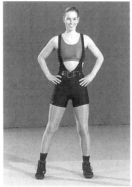 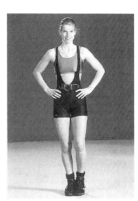

Step Touch

Side to Side (or also Plié Touch or Side Tip)   *2 beats*

Weight is transferred to the side from the basic starting position and the legs are opened a little further. The tip of the foot of the active leg taps the ground. Weight transfer follows after standing on the ball of one's foot on the load-bearing leg.

Correct performance:

- Knee joint of the stationary leg always remains slightly bent and still and does not bounce.
- Heel of the stationary leg remains on the ground and does not bounce.
- Pelvis and upper body are kept facing forwards.

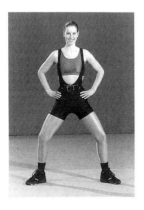 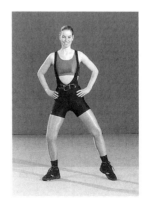

Hopscotch (or Hamstring Curl or Leg Curl)   *2 beats*

Weight transfer from the basic position to the side as in Side to Side. Foot of the active leg does not tap the ground but is moved towards one's bottom by bending the knee joint. At the same time the lower leg is raised into an almost horizontal position.

Correct performance:

- Knee joint of the stationary leg always remains slightly bent, is still and does not bounce.
- Heel of the stationary leg remains on the ground and does not bounce.
- Distance between the knees remains the same throughout.

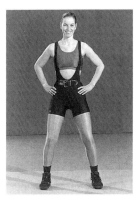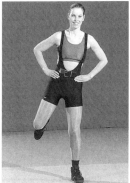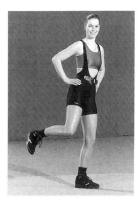

Hopscotch

Knee Lift (or also Knee Up)   *2 beats*

A leg is bent with no weight stress and then lifted forwards, until the knee is at approximately the same height as the hip. This step is also often done in a high-impact version (jumped).

Correct performance:

- The stationary leg always remains slightly bent.
- The knee is only raised about as far as hip level (danger of shifting in the vertebral column tilting the upper body forward).
- Knee joint of the stationary leg remains still and slightly bent.

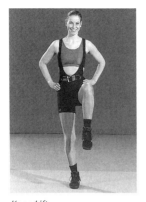

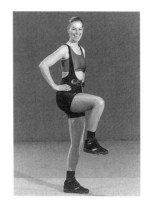

Knee Lift
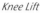

Heel Dig (or also Heel Touch)   2 beats

Both legs are slightly bent and the active leg is stretched out straight forwards or diagonally forwards, whilst the heel of the stationary leg is on the ground.

Correct performance:

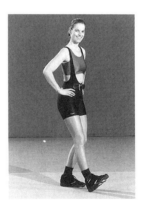

- Knee joint of the stationary leg remains still.
- Knee joint of the stationary leg always remains behind the tip of the foot (do not bend too much).

Lunge (Falling Forward Step)   2 beats

Lunges can be done in various ways. The lunge movement of the leg can, for example, be done backwards, diagonally backwards, to the side or forwards. At the same time the lunging leg can be bent (flexed lunges) or stretched. Perhaps we should explain just two variations of this step which is technically very demanding.

Both legs are slightly bent, then the active leg is stretched out backwards, the ball of the foot touches the ground and the leg has weight put onto it.

At the same time the body weight is obviously transferred from the stationary leg backwards, whilst the upper body compensates by moving forwards slightly.

In the variation the active leg is stretched out diagonally backwards; then one must turn so far, balanced on the ball of the foot of the stationary leg, that the stationary and lunging leg as well as the upper body are all in line with each other.

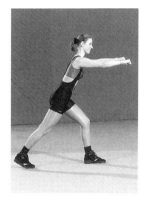

Lunge

In order to learn the movement correctly, it is recommended to slow down to half temper (four beats per movement).

Correct performance:

• Heel to the lunging leg remains in the air.
• The lunging leg remains stretched.
• The knee joint of the stationary leg remains behind the tip of the foot.
• The axis of foot, knee, hip, upper body is maintained.

Grapevine *4 beats*

The first step is diagonally to the side, whereby the foot is rolled from the heel to the ball of one's foot and then has weight put on it. The free leg is crossed over behind and then weight is transferred to the crossed-over leg. Both of the following steps (movements) match the movements of Step Touch.

Correct performance:

• The first step to the side is done with the heel.
• Upper body and pelvis remain facing forwards throughout the whole movement.
• Upper body remains upright.
• Knee joints always remain slightly bent, but do not give way (especially when crossed over backwards).

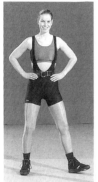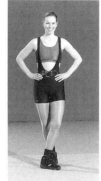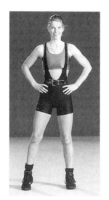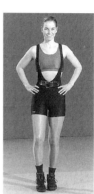

Grapevine

Mambo   *4 beats*

Mambo is a variation on Marching, during which one leg performs a marching movement with the other leg alternately somewhat further forwards like a rolling movement in Walking, and then slightly behind the body. The high-impact version of this step is called Rock Step.

Correct performance:

- Knee joints remain slightly bent.
- Upper body remains upright.

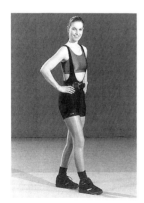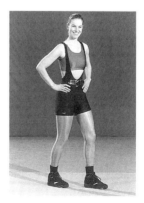

Mambo

Pivot Turn   *4 beats*

The pivot turn can easily be developed from a Mambo. The right foot is set down forwards and rolled from the heel. Finally, half a turn is done to the left on the balls of both feet. The right foot is put down again forwards and rolled off, finishing with another half turn to the left on the balls of the feet. In this movement pattern the left foot remains still and the right foot revolves round it.

    If the left foot leads, the turning happens the other way round and the right remains still.

Correct performance:

- The turning is done on the balls of the feet.
- The turning follows on from setting down and rolling off the leading leg.
- The upper body remains upright.

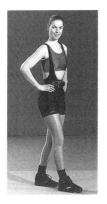 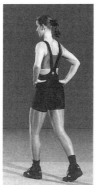 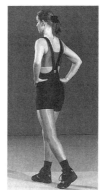 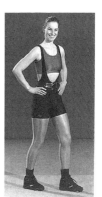

Pivot Turn

Jogging (or also Jog = Running)   *2 beats*

Whilst running on the spot the feet are rolled away from the balls of the feet to the heels. The lower legs are raised to about knee height and the arms swung in a slightly bent position alternately and rhythmically.

Correct performance:

- Each setting down of the foot implies a rolling away to the heel.

Low Kick   *2 beats*

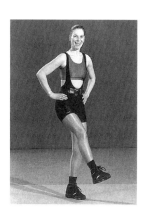

One leg is stretched out forwards, stretching the foot as well. The stationary leg completes a small hopping movement (hop) at the same time.

The stretched-out leg is then brought to the stationary leg, which does another hop (high-impact variation). In the low-impact variation the hops are omitted.

The kicking leg can also be brought forward diagonally to the side or streched out backwards.

Correct performance:

- The stationary leg remains bent.
- The kicking leg is taken away from the body in a controlled movement.
- The upper body remains upright.

Jumping Jack   *2 beats*

Both legs are opened by jumping, and the feet, significantly further apart than hip width, are then brought back to the ground. At the same time knees and feet are slightly turned outwards and the knee joints slightly bent, so that the jump can be cushioned.

The feet are again rolled off from the balls to the heels on landing. During a second jump the legs are closed again with feet parallel. The same principle applies to putting the feet down as in the opening movement.

Correct performance:

- Knees and feet are turned outwards slightly on opening.
- The feet are rolled off at every jump, from the balls of the feet to the heels.
- The legs are opened far enough for the knee joints by bending to remain behind the tips of the feet when cushioning a jump.

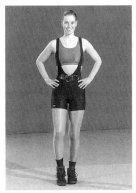 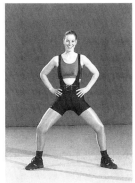 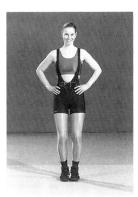

Jumping Jack

Scoop   *2 beats*

Scoop is a high-impact variation of Step Touch. One leg, as in Step Touch, is set out to the side and has weight put on it. Then a closing jump is done and both feet are rolled off from the balls to the heels.

Correct performance:

- Knee joints always remain slightly bent.
- Feet are closed after the jump.

Squat   *4 beats*

During a squat, bending the knee joints is combined with bending one's trunk, so that the upper body is brought forwards. During all of these movements, even weight balance is maintained across the entire soles of one's feet (body's centre of gravity remains above the feet). To achieve this one's bottom must be brought back a long way and the knee joints always remain behind the tips of the feet. The feet can either be placed apart in line with the hips (parallel legs), or set further apart from each other (legs turned outwards slightly).

In both versions take care that the knee joints always point in the direction of the tips of the feet.

The not-so-well trained should take the weight off their back by supporting themselves on the thighs above the knee-caps.

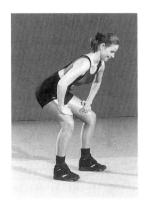 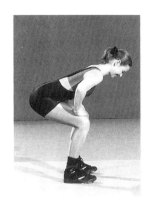

Squat

4.1.4 Arm Movements

With arm movements the conceptual variety is infinitely more confusing than with step patterns. Very few arm movements have the same descriptions, many of which have been taken into aerobic sport from the areas of strength training/dumb-bell training. Some of the most common are introduced below.

The following principle applies to all movement patterns: a neutral position of the wrists is maintained i.e. the wrists are neither bent excessively nor overstretched. The fingers can easily be curled into the fist.

Biceps Curl

Both elbows are fixed firmly against the sides of the body, and in the starting position the arms are almost stretched with the palms of the hands facing forwards (thumb to the outside). The elbow joints are bent and stretched. In the final position the palms of the hands are turned towards the body (thumbs outwards again).

In a variation the lower arms are turned during the bending. Starting position: palms of the hand towards each other (thumbs forwards), closing position (bent elbow joints) is as above.

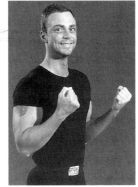
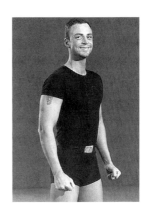

Biceps Curl

Triceps Kickback (or Triceps Curl)

In the starting position the arms are taken behind the back, elbow joints bent and hands towards the front. During the movement the elbows remain fixed behind the body with the palms of the hands facing each other. The elbow joints are now stretched and bent, taking care that the elbow joints are not overstretched in the final position.

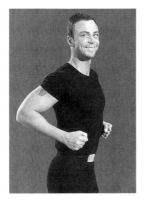
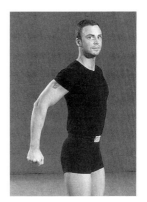

Triceps Kickback

Upright Row (or Shoulder Row up or Vertical Rowing)

In the starting position the arms are almost stretched out beside the body with the palms of the hands facing backwards (thumbs pointing inwards).

During the movement the arms are raised, elbow joints bent and then raised sideways to the same level as the shoulders, with the hands towards the shoulders in the final position.

Watch that the shoulders are not raised.

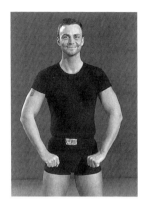

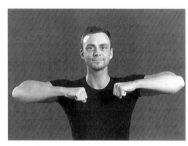

Upright Row

Front Arm Raise (or Front Laterals or Front Lifting)

In the starting position the arms are almost stretched out to lie at the side of the body, with the palms of the hands pointing backwards. The arms now complete an opposite version (the arms are raised in front of the body) until elbows and hands reach the same level as the shoulders. It is important here that the arms are not overstretched at the elbow joints, and that they are not raised higher than the shoulders or thrown forwards.

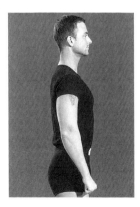

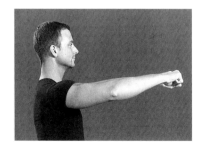

Front Laterals

Lateral Arm Raise (Side Laterals or Lifting Sideways)

In the starting position the arms are again placed at the side of the body, almost stretched, with the palms of the hands facing each other. The arms are raised so far sideways that elbows and hands are at the same level as the shoulders, taking care that the arms are not raised further than shoulder-level.

A variation on this movement is to do it with the elbows bent at right angles.

Chest Press

To start with the hands are in front of the shoulders with the elbows at shoulder-level. The arms are now stretched at chest-height away from the body with the palms of the hands pointing downwards, ensuring that the elbow joints are not overstretched and remain level with the shoulders.

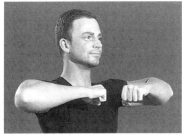
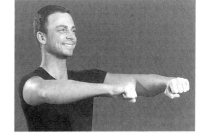

Chest Press

Overhead Press (or Neck Shoulder Press) (or Neck Press)

The arms start in the same position as for Chest Press. Then the arms are stretched above the head with the palms of the hands pointing forwards. The movement is not done vertically upwards, but rather slightly towards the front, taking care that the elbow joints are not overstretched.

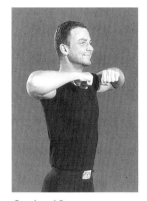

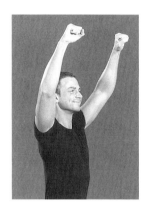

Overhead Press

Butterfly

The elbows are bent at right angles to the side of the body at shoulder-level, with the lower arms upright into the air and palms facing each other. The lower arms are now brought round in front of the body with elbows at chest level and palms pointing inwards. The elbows should not be lowered too far during this movement.

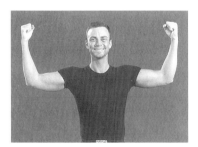

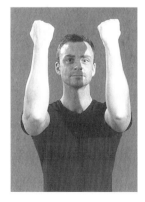

Butterfly

4.2 Music and Movement

Aerobics is a kind of movement to music i.e. all patterns of movement are adapted to music and the music dictates the tempo.

Well-chosen music creates the right atmosphere in each phase of the aerobics class and is the basic motivating force for the participants, as it increases the desire to make more effort or fosters relaxation.

4.2.1 Basic Structures of Music

Beat and Rhythm

The beat is what one often involuntarily taps out with one's hand or foot (e.g. percussion or bass). In between two beats is the "off-beat". Normal movement patterns in an aerobics class emphasise the beat i.e. they follow it, but sometimes, for example, "funk-aerobics" concentrates on the "off-beat".

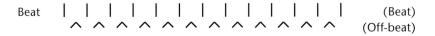

Beat | | | | | | | | | | | | | (Beat)
          ∧ ∧ ∧ ∧ ∧ ∧ ∧ ∧ ∧ ∧ ∧ ∧   (Off-beat)

In modern pop music the down-beat is emphasised more than the up-beat:

	2		4		6		8		Up-beat
Beat		1		3		5		7	Down-beat
Emphasis	▌				▌					▌				▌			

A movement begun on the down-beat often motivates more, and is easier to move to than one which starts on the up-beat.

For example, if you listen to a waltz and tap with the beat, you will notice that one beat is emphasised after which two beats have less emphasis. The emphasised beat is always counted as "1" and the two following beats as "2" and "3". This sequence of an emphasised beat and two unemphasised beats gives the typical waltz rhythm which we all know. Other dances (i.e. forms of music and movement) have other typical sequences of emphasised and unemphasised beats, that is to say, other rhythms.

Modern pop music is characterised by a typical sequence of emphasised and less-emphasised beats, whereby the first of eight beats is especially strong. With a bit of practice you can find this first beat in the music, which then helps the listening to the melody and the sung text.

Beat	1	2	3	4	5	6	7	8
Emphasis	■	'			'	■	'			'

Therefore, an aerobics trainer should, for safety's sake, and in time to the music, begin to introduce new step patterns or a combination of steps on a "1", as starting with "3" or "5" means working against the music.

Various types of fast music are used in the different phases of an aerobics class. The speed of the music is measured in beats per minute (bpm).

The following data are recommended music speeds:

Warming-up and cooling down phase	124-136 bpm
Cardio-phase	
Low-impact	128-152 bpm
High-impact	140-160 bpm
Mixed-impact	140-152 bpm
Floorwork	112-128 bpm
Stretching	slow and relaxing

We do not advise working below or above these limits due to subsequent reduced efficacy i.e. greater risk of injury.

Melody and Phrasing

The melody normally lies above the beat as a series of sounds of varying levels and duration. In modern pop music, if you listen carefully, you will notice that eight beats always belong close together because the subsequent melody is repeated in an exact or similar way, or a line of the text is sung exactly the same or similarly. Each of these sections with eight beats (emphasising the first) is called a phrase. The beginning of a phrase often coincides with the first emphasised of eight beats.

When one is experienced in feeling one's way into the beat of the music, one can often detect that four phrases, i. e. four times eight beats, belong close together musically. From time to time four phrases constitute a set or movement (also known as a musical curve). To fit in with this, permanent, complex combinations, aerobic movements are always planned in units of 32 (= 4 x 8) beats.

As far as aerobics trainers are concerned it would be good if all music was as clearly structured as just described, which is by no means always the case. In many songs there are "breaks" (also called "bridges"), which is a desired "accident" by the composer (as special effect) during the regular sequence of four phrases each containing eight beats, to which he adds a few beats. So, instead of 32 beats, the phrase may contain 36 or 40 beats.

As aerobic choreographies are always planned with a series of 32 beats (corresponding to the normal length of a phrase), the problem arises that the repeat choreography cannot always be started in tune with the musical structure as required.

For aerobic trainers with little practise in working with music, we recommend avoiding music with breaks. The good sort of cassettes specially compiled for aerobics lessons contain no breaks.

4.2.2 Music and Combinations of Steps

When trying to fit the aerobic step pattern perfectly in time with the music, one must ascertain how many beats are needed for the run-through of a basic step. Thus, for example, a Step Touch or Jumping Jack lasts for two beats, whereas a Grapevine or V-Step lasts four beats.

A combination of aerobic steps i.e. a permanent and repeatable series of movement patterns, comprises 32 beats or sets of 32 beats in line with the phrase (music curve) described above. Therefore, when lining up steps in a choreography one should always count exactly how many beats are needed for the steps already done, and how many steps must still follow to complete the movement correctly. For example, with 32 beats one could do:

2 Grapevines	= 8 beats
+ 4 Step Touches	= 8 beats
+ 2 V-Steps	= 8 beats
+ 4 Jumping Jacks	= 8 beats
combination of steps	= 32 beats

4.2.3 Counting to the Music

The simplest way of counting out loud to the music is with a number for each beat:

Beat									
Counting	1	2	3	4	5	6	7	8

One says that each beat has a corresponding "count".

This is not always the case. Under certain circumstances it is better to only have two or four beats per count:

Beat									
First type of counting	1	2	3	4	5	6	7	8	...
Second type of counting	1		2		3		4		...
Third type of counting	1				2				...

If the trainer is counting her participants into a new movement (Cueing see 4.3), she will not count the beats to the start, as this sequences would be too fast for the participants. Usually she would count the steps to be done before the start from "4" backwards, i.e. in Grapevines she puts four beats to one count, saying "Still 4 Grapevines, still 3, still 2, still 1", but in Step Touches she puts two beats to one count.

An aerobics trainer just beginning her training will find it difficult at first to count the music at the same time as doing the movement, planning the next movements and counting the participants into the next movement (counting in). Being able to synchronise these activities well is the mark of a good aerobics trainer. It becomes routine as experience in teaching increases.

4.2.4 Choice of Music

When choosing the music for an aerobics class, the trainer should aim to please most of her participants. So the use of certain types of music like Techno, House, Latin, Rock etc. is not to be recommended if the participants see it more as a disturbing noise screen rather than motivating their movements.

Depending on the phase of aerobics arrived at, one should vary the character of the music used. The music for warming-up should constitute a motivating introduction, but not encourage jumping movements or be too hectic. One should also carefully monitor the volume.

During the cardio-phase the music should drive on i.e. support the enjoyment of the movement.

When cooling down, on the other hand, the music should become calmer and, although at the same speed as when warming-up, should convey a feeling of relaxation. Perhaps a song with disguised Latin-American rhythm would be better suited to this rather than music with a strong beat.

For floorwork we recommend clearly-structured music with a clearly recognisable beat which promotes controlled muscular work. For the stretching part, one should use music specially designed for relaxing, which can create a quiet background for the exercises.

4.3 Cueing

Cueing describes the sum total of all linguistic and optical aids available to an aerobics trainer for giving the participants in training clear and unmistakable directions without interrupting the flow of training.

Cueing
(sum total of all linguistic and optical means)

- Unequivocal
- Timely
- Resolute/convincing (*not* hesistant)
- Aim: lesson runs without a break

Verbal Cueing	**Non-verbal Cueing**
• Linguistic cues • Tips • Motivation	• Body language • Facial expressions (e.g. smiling) • Gestures (e.g. head nodding) • Signs and symbols (e.g. international handsigns) "Visual preview"

Cueing comprises all the possibilities of **verbal** (linguistic) and **non-verbal** (non-linguistic) communication, which the aerobics trainer can employ. Verbal cueing allows for motivation, praise and criticism as well as directions and helpful positions. We list the most important elements of verbal cueing as follows:

- Description of the following pattern of movement.
- Direction about the starting foot.
- Direction for use of the arm.
- Indication of the direction of movement, turns etc.
- Indication of the tempo of the movement.
- A count of the number of repeats until changeover.
- Preparation for the participants.
- Possible corrective instructions.

For ease of linguistic communication radio-microphones are often used. These help the aerobic trainer in her work with larger groups, and in big rooms like a sports hall. As these high-quality radio-microphones, which continue to produce good tone quality despite being shaken by jumping movements, are still relatively expensive, they are not normally available for aerobics trainers.

However, it is important to note that whether one wants it or not, non-verbal messages are always part of the communication process. One's body language in facial expressions and gestures conveys what one really thinks and feels. The vocal combination of language on the one hand and non-verbal messages through body language etc. on the other hand, is vital when we wish to convey something effectively, according to psychologists.

In this case, all the visual signs and symbols, which the trainer uses in addition to verbal cueing in order to lead the aerobic group securely, have a particularly important role to play. This non-verbal cueing is a decided advantage when leading training, especially when the trainer can no longer be easily heard. Also it supports verbal cueing and confirms the fact that many people can be reached faster and better by optical than by acoustic (verbal) signals.

A prerequisite for working with signs is that they are introduced gradually and clearly and are confidently and consistently used. Because of the importance

"4 more"	"3 more" (1st possibility)	or "3 more" (2nd possibility)

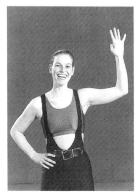 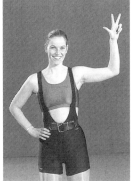 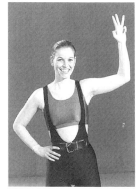

"2 more"

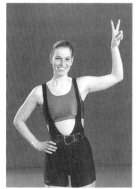

"1 more"

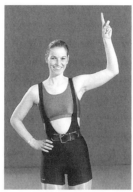

"March"

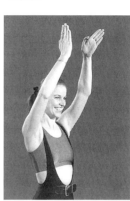

"Stop"
(Hold/Stay)

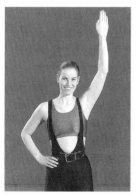

"From the beginning"
(From the top)

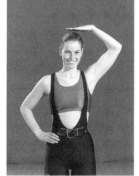

"Add Arms"

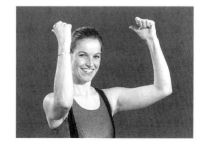

"Front"

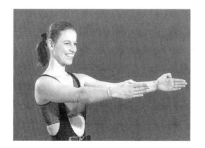

"Back"

"To the left"   *"To the right"*

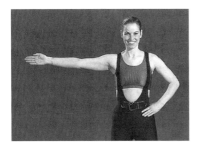 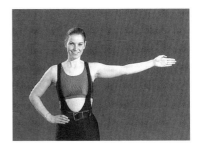

"Well done" (Good job)   *"Circle"*

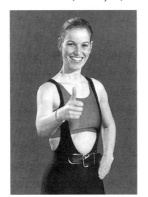 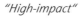 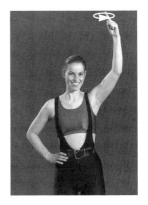

"Low-impact"   *"High-impact"*   *"Just watch, don't do it yet" (watch me)*

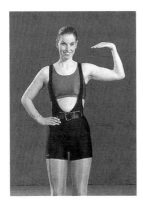 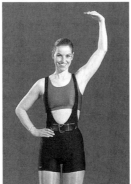 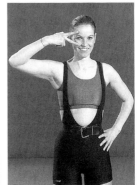

of visual signs for communication, one has been trying to find an international norm – the international hand signs – for some time:

One must ensure that cueing is quite unmistakable. Therefore, all directions must be totally clear and remain the same, so that every participant, whether in the front or back row, is clear which movement to do next.

Therefore, use the international hand signs and symbols all the time and not any you have invented yourself, because that could cause you big problems later when teaching an unknown group.

If you keep to the agreed international hand signs you can assume that you will be allowed to teach unhindered wherever these signs are used. So that the hand signs are clearly recognisable for each participant in the room, the cues must always be confidently, clearly and speedily given above head height. If the trainer gives the directions in front of her body they will reach the participants in the first two rows, but be of little use to those in the back rows.

Knowing when to introduce cueing is of paramount importance to its success. Therefore, all directions must follow on from one another at the correct time, so that each participant can prepare for the next movement i.e. whilst one movement is running the aerobics trainer must give loud and clear information about the following movement. Whilst doing this she should count out (4 more, 3 more, 2 more, 1 more) as well as non-verbally (with hand signs) cueing the participants into the next movement.

If interruptions occur in the training unit, because the participants cannot follow the aerobics trainer, then the cueing should be analysed first. Mistakes found most often in cueing are when they are given too late i.e. that cueing is certainly given, but too late for the participants to understand in the brief remaining time before the next movement pattern, let alone put it into action (e.g. 4 more, 3 more, 2 more, Grapevine). Another mistake which crops up frequently is an incomprehensible cueing, i.e. the cueing comes in time, but so unclearly that the participants do not know what to do next (e.g. speaking too quietly when cueing, or unclear non-standardised hand signs/hand signs straight out in front of one's body).

Another way of teaching step patterns is to demonstrate the movement, without the participants' taking part. This kind of teaching method gives the participants an visual workout of a potentially complex step pattern.

The announcement of a "visual preview" follows with the hand-sign "watch me". This sort of hand-sign is a very common additional aid when used sparingly.

Important and indispensible as good cueing is, please ensure that you do not overdo your cueing. Unnecessary repeating of instructions, monotonous or overemphasised announcements, disturb the participants and the proceedings. As the use of cueing is so indispensible for the smooth running of an aerobics class, and because it is vital to the participants' motivation, you should study your cueing carefully and then use it with discretion in your aerobics classes.

4.4 Mirrored Working

Aerobics classes usually take place in rooms with one or two mirror walls, which enables the teacher to work with her back to the group. A good aerobics trainer can be recognised by the extent to which she has her face towards her participants. Normally, during work in sport halls there is no alternative to leading the training facing the group.

Direct contact with the group achieved by facing them is vital to creating a personal and motivating atmosphere, regardless of external conditions.

However, one is then forced to demonstrate all the movements to be carried out by the participants using the mirror, because only by mirroring the exercises during a demonstration, can the participants imitate them immediately, without having to think them first the other way round. Finally, it is important that the participants concentrate on the aerobics class and their own personal interpretation.

Of course a mirrored lesson is not easy initially, and it requires some practice to get used to it. During this "trial run" you should constantly remember the advantages of teaching facing the group.

- Communication between trainer and group is more direct and more personal.
- The participants can understand the trainer's directions much better, because the voice resonance travels forwards, where the group is in front of you.

- The trainer can react faster and better to any uncertainty in performing the movements than if she were to have her back to the group.
- The trainer can also keep an eye on the well-being of her participants (heart-circulation problems, training too intensively etc), than when everything takes place "behind her back", so to speak.

Another feature of mirrored work is in the turns. Turns are first done not facing the group. Once the participants have got the hang of the turn after two or three demonstrations, the aerobics trainer turns to face the group and does the turn the other way round i.e. the participants turn to the right, for example, and the aerobics trainer to the left.

As you can see, there are many advantages in mirrored work, as it is easily learnt and should be part of every aerobics trainer's repertoire.

PRACTICAL TIPS AND INSTRUCTIONS

The participants march on the right foot i.e. to each "1", they lift their right foot, to "2" their left foot, to "3" their right foot again etc.	The aerobics trainer marches on the left foot i.e. to each "1", she lifts the left foot, to "2" the right foot, to "3" the left foot again etc, i.e. the opposite way round to her participants.
The participants should complete a pattern of steps to the right, starting on the right foot.	The aerobics trainer must do the pattern of steps (as seen by her) to the left, starting on the left foot.
The participants should complete a step pattern forwards, starting on the right foot.	The aerobics trainer must do the pattern of steps (as seen by her) backwards, starting on the left foot.
Exception: The participants should do a V-step, starting on the right foot.	Exception: This is a step pattern, where the two first steps are done forwards, so the trainer also does her first two steps forwards, towards the group and starting on the left foot. Likewise: Mambo

5 Phases of an Aerobics Class

5.1 Overview

The structure of an aerobics class is directed towards the main aim of aerobic training, which is to improve one's endurance potential i.e. oxygen absorption capacity. In addition to this, other fitness components are trained in an aerobics class (strength, flexibility, co-ordination) and this is reflected to varying degrees depending on the aim of that lesson.

The general structure of an aerobics class comprises five main phases:
• Warming-up
• Cardio-phase
• Cooling down
• Floorwork
• Stretching

Warming-up

As in all training units an aerobics class begins with a warming-up phase, the aim of which is to prepare the body for the following physical stress by raising the body's basic temperature, by a slowly-increasing pulse rate and by the stimulation of the production of synovial fluid (see 3.1.1). These processes must be set in motion slowly, to avoid risk of injury. The music speed is about 124-136 bpm. The length of time taken to warm up should be about 15% of the total length of the lesson i.e. ten minutes of a 60 minute lesson.

Cardio-phase

This phase lies at the "heart" of an aerobics class, and it aims to improve one's endurance potential (capacity to absorb oxygen) by slightly reduced stress (60-85% of the maximum pulse rate) is achieved over a sufficiently lengthy period of time (15-30 minutes). Here also we adhere to the principle that changing the speed of the music (and thus also the stress) must not happen suddenly, but slowly. During the first few minutes of a cardio-phase (pre-aerobics) the intensity increases successively, but then remains for a while in a steady state and falls away again slowly (post-aerobics). This intensity curve is regulated by step and movement patterns of varying levels of intensity, and also the music's speed (low-impact: 128-158 bpm; high/low-impact: 140-160 bpm).

Cooling down

During cooling down, the heart and circulation processes are stabilised. By slowly reducing the intensity of movement sequences (slight radius, small leverage), the pulse rate is lowered and a possible collection of blood in one's lower extremities avoided. The music speed should be about 124-136 bpm. A slight turning of the main muscles used in the cardio-phase (m. gastrocnemius, m. soleus, ischiocrural muscles) at the end of cooling down prevents injury. Cooling down should last about five minutes.

Floorwork

The aim of floorwork is to strengthen all the body muscles (increasing muscular strength and endurance of muscular strength). Special attention is given to groups of muscles which have not been trained adequately in the previous phase of the aerobics class, and also muscle groups which are inclined to be weaker for various reasons (outer upper thigh, bottom, tummy, back), and so one gains better control of one's movements and a healthier body posture. As the various muscle groups should be trained separately (i.e. without any assistance from supporting muscles), many of the movements are done lying on the floor. The music speed should be chosen sufficiently carefully (112-128 bpm) for the movements to be done vigorously and without any jumping. This whole phase should last 10-15 minutes.

Stretching

In the final phase of the aerobics class muscles, which have been used in the previous phases should be stretched in order to avoid contraction of these muscle groups, and to thus prevent injury. A basic improvement in one's flexibility should be attained via this aspect of injury prevention. The music should create a feeling of physical and mental relaxation, and at least 5-10 minutes is envisaged for this phase of the aerobics class.

5.2 Warming-up

5.2.1 General Aims

During the warming-up phase the body should be prepared carefully for the physical stress to come. The all-round physical preparation to perform should be increased and adapted to the amount of exercise required by activitating the heart and circulatory system, and adapting the muscle and joint metabolism.

One can thus avoid injury to the active and passive mobility system, as well as avoiding signs of reduced potential like premature tiredness etc.

5.2.2 Specific Effects of Warming-up

Effects on the Muscle Structure

By using as many of the larger groups of muscles as possible one can increase warmth, and the muscle temperature is consequently raised. The body's basic temperature can also be raised by channelling warmth into the centre of the body via the blood. A range between 38,5 and 39 C° is seen to be best. An increase in the body's basic temperature ensures a kind of counter-move, in that it stabilises the muscle temperature.

Certain metabolic processes (i.e. enzyme activities) important to physical performance run best at these raised temperatures.
Any superfluous heat is shed through the skin to the outside i.e. the one begins to sweat.
The elasticity of the warmed-up muscles improves visibly, and any impeding influences against contraction i.e. stretching the muscles whilst working, are reduced, thus also reducing danger of injury.

Consequently, strength, speed and ability to maintain muscle contraction all increase.

The muscles and the skin have their blood supply increased by the opening and widening of the capillaries, so that oxygen and energy-giving substances are delivered more effectively, and so that carbondioxide and other metabolic products can be taken away better.

Effects on the Heart and Circulatory System

To enable the transport system to do justice to the increased demands of the muscular metabolism, the amount of blood being carried in the working muscles is drastically increased per unit of time. This is achieved primarily by a higher pulserate, but also the amount of blood in the heart chamber, emitted at each heart beat, is increased (increase in the amount of blood output by stronger contractions of the heart).

Overall, the heart-time-volume is increased (= pulse rate x amount per beat).

On the other hand, the blood circulation through kidneys and stomach-gut area is reduced, and a recirculation of the blood takes place.

Also the breath-time-volume (= breathing rate x amount per breath) increases i.e. for each time unit. The working muscle receives more oxygen by faster and deeper breathing (breath frequency and amount per breath). More oxygen can be absorbed per breath, and the amount of oxygen taken in per breath, which is then actually used by the muscles, is increased.

By raising the blood temperature, consolidated amounts of oxygen can be delivered to the working muscles more efficiently.

One's systolic blood pressure rises (indicating heart performance), but the diastolic rate remains more or less constant (indicating the elasticity of the artery walls).

Effects on the Joints

Even joint structures adapt to the increased demands of physical stress. By alternately stressing and relaxing the joints as well as from the movement in the joints, more synovial fluid is produced, and so friction between areas of cartilage is less. To a certain extent synovial fluid is pressed into the cartilage which sucks itself full and thus becomes fatter. In this way, unwanted pressure can be warded off better.

The elasticity of various ligaments is increased by a rise in temperature.

Effects on the Conduction of Impulses

When one's temperature is raised, the sensitivity of the sense receptors in skin, muscles and tendons rises, and with it one's co-ordinating performance ability, because these measuring sensors give important data for the accuracy of movements to the central nervous system. The increased temperature also leads to an improvement in the conducting of nerve impulses and thus to an improved speed of conduction.

The increased sensitivity of the central nervous system also causes a greater speed of reaction and contraction in the muscles.

Effects on the Psychological and Mental Area

The warming-up procedure activitates certain areas of the brain, apparent from a state of increased wakefulness i.e. improved powers of perception and optical awareness. In addition, the participants improve their self-confidence and build up trust in their trainer. The participants attention is transferred from the demands of everyday life to the sporting exertion. One can create an pleasant atmosphere, fun and pleasurable anticipation with appropriate types of movement and skillfull communication between trainer and participants.

5.2.3 Warming-up for an Aerobics Lesson

Raising the muscle and body temperature on which, as already described, many positive effects relating to the body's preparation for stress depend, is attained by doing whole-body movements. These are movements in which both arms and legs are involved, so that as large an amount of all the body's muscles as possible is used. Therefore, it makes sense, to begin with, to perform consistently smaller and less intensive movements and then to gradually increase the stress. The intensity of a movement is thereby especially dependent on the size of the muscles used and the movement's radius.

The optimum amount of stress for warming-up puts high demands on the trainer and calls for experience and the ability to empathize. Too intensive a warming-up time leads to overacidity in the working muscles, and the participants already feel tired after warming-up. On the other hand, with too little intensity in the warming-up phase, the likelihood of having a positive effect on the heart and circulatory system, muscles and joints is put in jeopardy.

The content of the movement programme should be aimed towards movement patterns occurring later in the stress phase.

For the joints to receive the best kind of preparation, one should establish that they can be moved within a suitable large, functional radius, just right for them, and in a fluent, smooth performance over a large period of time. We make particular mention here of the knee joints, shoulder joints and ankle joints, which have a particularly sensitive anatomical structure and are put under a wide variety of pressure in an aerobics class.

Towards the end of a warming-up phase, muscles which are to receive greater stress later are often statically or dynamically prestretched i.e. they are stretched carefully and only briefly. This procedure clearly differs in its timespan and intensity, and thus also in its effect from stretching muscles after physical stress. The specific aim of this prestretching during warming-up is a controversial issue in sports science, and its value in aerobics classes in the area of leisure and general sport is increasingly questionable.

In order to maintain the pulse rate and muscle temperature once they have been reached, this part of warming-up is kept short, that is, the pre-stretches are kept separate by whole-body movements in between times.

Especially the calf muscles, the leg-bending and hip-bending muscles, as well as the chest and shoulder muscles can be prestretched in this way.

5.2.4 The Practical Setting-up of a Warming-up Phase

The aerobics trainer can put many different movement patterns into the warming-up phase. The following list is intended to help a little in one's choice. When selecting a combination of movements, one should ensure that they can flow smoothly and harmoniously into each other.

One often starts in a basic position with legs slightly apart, knee joints bent a little and with gentle circling of the shoulders (a more static variation), or with marching (a more dynamic variation).

Suitable Step Patterns

Marching/Walking (on the spot, forwards, backwards, to the outside, to the inside etc.), V-Step, Side to Side, Push Touch, Hopscotch, Knee Lift, Heel Dig, Plié.

Non-recommended Step Patterns

- High-impact step patterns (no jogging or anything similar!). The stress on joint structures (and spine) is disproportionally much too high.
- Complicated, lateral movement patterns like Grapevine, Side gallop or Cha Cha. When doing Grapevine the trainer should estimate whether the step already presents most of the participants with a high degree of co-ordination, or whether the step has already become automatic and its use could be risked.
- Low-impact movement patterns with obviously more stress on the joints than desired e.g. Lunges. The knee joint and Achilles' tendon are put under

extreme pressure if this exercise is done incorrectly. Also the stress on heart and circulation can be undesirably high.
- Step patterns containing sudden turns or turns stressful for the knee joints.

Suitable Arm Movements

In order to prepare the joints and muscles fully, one should aim to work with as much variety as possible. Begin with smaller movements with short leverage (bent elbow joints), and then, later, longer levers and movements with a large radius can be employed. Various levels of movement should alternate and the movements flow into each other harmoniously. Arm movements above the head should only be carried out carefully and on no account at the start of warming-up

Arm Movements Non-recommended

Dynamically executed circling movements in the shoulder joint and with a long lever (outstretched arm) and large radius of movement can make it difficult for the shoulder joint to function, especially when the arm is pulled back behind the body at the same time. Small, fast movements with long levers put just as much stress on the shoulder joints.

Moving through the Joints (Joint Isolation)

Shoulder-blade/shoulder joints:
- Pull up the shoulders.
- Circle the shoulders.
- front lift, sideways lift, Butterfly, Chest Press etc.
- Circling movements in the shoulder joint.

Ankle joints:
- Heels remain on the ground, foot is pulled up and set down again (without taxing the leg if possible).
- Balls of the feet remain on the ground, heel is lifted and put down again (e.g. in an easy step position).

Knee joints:
- Hopscotch
- Knee Lift
- Plié.

Hip joints:
- Knee Lift
- Lift leg to the side
- Plié.

Spinal column:
* Bend the trunk forwards, supporting oneself on the thighs and, with legs bent, bend and stretch one's back.

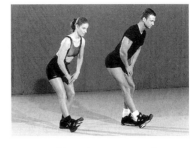

Prestretches

Which muscles are prestretched depend on the content of the stress phase. In a gymnastics class, with the emphasis on upperbody strengthening (inserting of Heavy Hands), other prestretches are done than during a class with many high-impact elements. Here now a few frequently-used stretching positions:

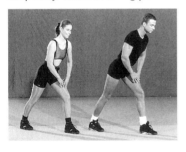

Leg-bending Muscles (Ischiocrural Muscles)

Tips for body posture:
* Back remains stretched.
* Head remains in line with the spine.
* Pelvis is not turned.
* Supporting oneself is done on the bent stationary leg.

Calf Muscles (M. Gastrocnemius)

Tips for body posture:
* Upper body is in extension of the line of the rear leg.
* Pelvis does not turn.
* Rear foot is not turned out.
* The feet do not stand directly behind each other (unstable!), but a little apart.
* Supporting oneself is done on the thighs, not the knee-caps.

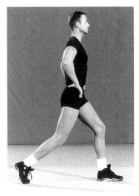

Hip-bender (M. Iliopsoas)

Tips for body posture:
* Upper body remains upright.
* Both legs are bent.
* Heel of rear foot stays in the air.
* Feet do not stand directly behind each other, but slightly apart.

Back-stretcher (M. Erector Spinae)

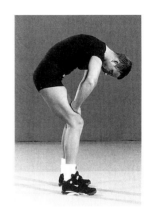

Tips for body posture:
* Both legs are clearly bent.
* Neck vertebrae are not overstretched.
* Supporting oneself is done on the thighs, not on the knee-caps.
* Fingers point at each other or forwards during the supporting.

The prestretches should not be done until towards the end of the warming-up phase, when the muscles have been warmed up, and they should be kept separate from whole-body movements to maintain the raised pulse rate.

5.2.5. Measuring the Amount of Warming-up

During the warming-up phase, the body should be prepared for the following exertion with a gradual increase in basic body temperature. Thus it should be capable of peak performance, but not already be tired. One should keep careful watch over this when gauging the stress intensity because working too hard during the warming-up phase leads to overacidity and tiredness in the working muscles. One should also decide, depending on the participants' level of fitness, which exercise can be used. For example, if knee-bending is used when training beginners, this can create a much too intensive strengthening stimulus, which is undesirable when warming-up.

One can only give a rough guide to the optimum length of the warming-up phase, because it is dependent on so many factors. One usually recommends about ten minutes at a time, during which the following should be observed:

* *Fitness Level of the Participants*
15-20 minutes of warming-up can be much too long and tiring for beginners if the total length of the training unit is perhaps around 30 minutes.

* *Age*
When training with senior citizens, one should be aware that raising the speed of metabolism towards increased performance potential takes more time. Warming-up should be done more slowly and carefully in order to prepare the less-elastic muscles and metabolically sluggish joint structures carefully.

• *Time of Day*
During a morning class one should warm up more carefully and longer than during an evening class, as certain body functions (like blood circulation through the muscles and basic body temperature) are greatly reduced whilst asleep, and do not reach their peak values until later in the day.

In addition to this, one's physiological performance potential varies during the course of the day, and is greater in the early evening than around two o'clock in the afternoon.

• *Surrounding Temperature*
If the surrounding temperature is too high this can lead to a reduction in warming-up time; low temperatures on the other hand (like cold sports halls) lengthen it.

5.3 Cardio-phase

5.3.1 General Aims

The cardio-phase constitutes the main part of a classic aerobics class and should last at least 15-30 minutes. Depending on the total length of the training unit, the cardio part can take a bit longer. One should aim at as long a cardio-phase as possible, because burning up the fat does not really get going properly until after about 20 minutes.

The speed of the music in the cardio part fits in with the style of aerobics being used at the time. For purely low-impact classes the music speed should be about 128-152 bpm. For high-low-impact classes the speed can reach up to 160 bpm; but if the number of beats is higher it is no longer possible to work in a technically accurate way, with the result that the intensity sinks and the risk of injury rises.

The prime aim of the cardio part is to improve the heart and circulation potential, by which one means the level of resistance of one's heart and circulatory system to tiredness.

Secondary aims are, on the one hand, an improvement in the composition of one's body. If one trains regularly and eats healthily in line with sporting principles, then one's body composition improves, i.e. the amount of fats decreases in favour of fat-free materials. On the other hand, the cardio part serves to improve one's neuro-muscular co-ordination. In aerobics training one concentrates first and foremost on exercises to improve one's exact co-ordination as much as co-ordination of the arms and legs.

In addition to this, the motoric memory is trained in an aerobics class whose cardio part is choreographied. Our motoric memory is responsible for our taking note of movements as far as very complex sequences (choreographies), and then being able to perform them in line with what we have seen.

Finally, one must not forget the motivational aspect: the enjoyment of movement. Naturally there are often good reasons why many adults only try out an aerobics class for a while, be it for fitness, one's figure or for one's health. If one cannot convey some sense of enjoyment in movement to participants, then they will not keep coming in the long term. The importance of motivation is addressed more thoroughly in chapter 9.

5.3.2 The Cardio-phase as Endurance Training

To do justice to endurance training from a preventative point of view, it is vital to get hold of a few scientific training principles. Firstly, that there simply is not just endurance training, but that the area of endurance is divided up as follows:

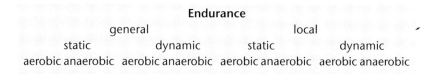

Endurance training in the cardio part of an aerobics class is concerned with training the general, aerobic, dynamic muscular endurance, or also basic endurance. The terms "general" and "local" tell us something about the range of the working muscles. If one is talking about general muscle endurance, then one means that more than $1/7 - 1/6$ of the whole muscle structure must be used. Both of the expressions "aerobic" and "anaerobic" tell us something about the way in which energy is released, whereby aerobic means that the energy release occurs when oxygen is being used up. "Dynamic" and "static" describe the way in which the muscles work, and in dynamic muscle work there is a change from contraction to relaxation.

Endurance Method and Steady State

For endurance training to reach the desired levels of adaptation, the way in which one trains is particularly important. During the cardio-phase of a classic aerobics lesson one usually works with the endurance method (exception: interval training).

The cardio-phase can be divided into three: pre-aerobics, steady state and post-aerobics.

In the pre-aerobics phase, which only lasts a few minutes, the intensity should be increased slowly, so that the body can gradually prepare for the impending stress. Whatever you do do not do high-impact movements at this stage.

During steady state the use of oxygen by the muscles and absorption of oxygen by breathing should be kept in balance as long as possible by correct intensity control (lactate production = lactate reduction). If the intensity is not controlled well at this stage it can lead to the muscles' being worked so intensively that not enough oxygen can be absorbed by breathing. As a result the training becomes anaerobic, and more lactate (lactic acid) is produced than can simultaneously be reduced, so that the muscles overacidify. This can lead to the loading phase being stopped.

The post-aerobic phase only lasts a few minutes, whilst the heart and circulation stress is reduced, after which comes cooling down.

5.3.3 Measuring and Controlling Intensity

As well as putting stress on the heart and circulatory system, the skeletal muscles are also strained during endurance exertion exercise. The more strain put on the heart and circulatory system, the greater the muscles' need for oxygen. The correct parameter for measuring the intensity of this is actually the maximum capacity for oxygen absorption (VO_2 max.)

Maximum Oxygen Absorption (VO_2max)

The VO_2max. is the norm for defining the supply of oxygen (breathing), oxygen transportation (heart and circulation) and use of oxygen (muscle cells) during endurance training. To a certain extent it is the "overall criterion for one's endurance capacity", and indicates how much energy can be made

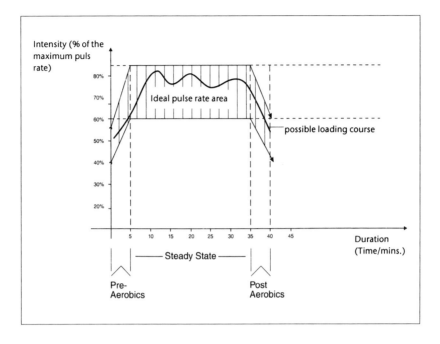

available aerobically over a specific length of time. Two measurements are necessary for calculating the VO_2max.: the volume per minute through the heart (i.e. the bonding capacity of oxygen in the blood), and the oxygen differential in the veins and arteries. The VO_2 max. reaches its highest level between 14 and 19 years of age. If no regular aerobic training is done then this level gradually sinks, but with aerobic training it is possible to maintain one's oxygen absorption capacity, that is delay its decline.

Lactate/Lactic Acid

Basically one can differentiate between two sorts of releasing energy: aerobic and anaerobic supply.

To assess the lasting potential of aerobics, one should assess the lactate level before, during, and after physical exercise as the most reliable criterion, because the blood's lactate concentration changes with the slightest alteration in performance.

Threshold levels help to define one's performance potential with the aid of lactate concentration in the blood: whilst the lactate concentration is between 1-1.78 mmol/l lactate when the body is at rest, the aerobic level reaches about 2 mmol/l lactate. This aerobic threshold indicates the limit of purely aerobic release of energy, i.e. lactate produced thus far eliminates itself again in the working muscle. Lactate production and lactate reduction are balanced out. During any further intense exercise, the anaerobic part of energy-release rises and with it also lactate production.

To a certain extent the lactate can be reduced by using up oxygen (aerobically). The threshold where that is still possible is around 2-4 mmol/l lactate. The threshold at which lactate production and reduction still balance each other is known as the aerobic-anaerobic threshold.

If training increases in intensity after this then it is no longer possible to reduce the level of lactic acid which then causes overacidity of the muscle, and consequently overtiredness.

This implies the following for aerobics training: a level of intense exercise should be reached during the cardio-phase, which is at the aerobic-anaerobic threshold level i.e. so that lactate production and reduction are balanced out (see steady state). If one works too intensively and oversteps the aerobic-anaerobic threshold, then the affected participant must stop the cardio-part.

Optimum Training Pulse Rate

Basically one can differentiate between three types of pulse rate: resting pulse, maximum pulse and training pulse.

The resting pulse is taken before one gets up in the morning and varies according to age and sex. It is also influenced by one's digestion, mental activity and the surrounding temperature, one's bio-rhythm, the general state of one's body and fitness level. The resting pulse is about 60 to 80 beats per min., which can be considerably lowered, if one is in training, without seeking a medical diagnosis.

Maximum pulse is the absolute highest biological pulse rate which anyone can have. The following rule-of-thumb helps you to calculate it:

220 minus one's age = maximum pulse (bpm)

The training pulse is the recommended pulse rate for aerobic endurance training. To calculate one's training pulse there are some useful formulae. A rough guide for untrained people is:

180 minus one's age = training pulse (bpm)

Because all participants are not at the same level of training, there is a somewhat more accurate formula which is often used for practical reasons:

60% of the maximum pulse = training pulse (lower limit)

85% of the maximum pulse = training pulse (upper limit)

Untrained participants should work along the lower limit and trained people along the upper limit.

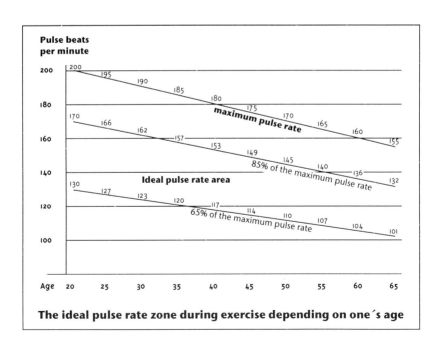

The ideal pulse rate zone during exercise depending on one´s age

Only when enough intensive training is done in the cardio-phase, is there enough stimulus for improving the endurance potential of heart and circulation, but, on the other hand, the intensity must be kept sufficiently low that enough oxygen for the aerobic release of energy to one's metabolism can take place. It is also important to observe the intensity of training of the participants, and if necessary, optimise the training.

One can measure intensity in one of three different ways: objective or subjective criteria, and someone else measuring you.

When measuring objectively one should assess one's use of oxygen, lactate concentration and pulse/heart rate. As it is impracticable to measure one's use of oxygen or lactate concentration during an aerobics class, one's training pulse is usually measured, although this is not such a reliable figure. One can take one's pulse by feeling the main arteries, at best by putting one's index and middle finger (not the thumb) on the radial artery or on the carotid artery.

Should the aerobics trainer wish to measure someone's pulse rate during the cardio part, then the music should be switched off. It is important to see that the participants keep moving, so that firstly there are no circulatory problems and, secondly, the training pulse is as accurate as possible. The pulse beats are taken for 15 seconds and then multiplied by 4 to obtain the pulse rate per minute (bpm). This result gives a rough guide, but with deviations of around 10-15 bpm because of the inaccuracy of such a method i.e. the aerobics trainer does not stop at exactly 15 seconds/the participants miscount/the pulse-rate falls again whilst being taken. However, even if a measurement is taken over a longer period of time i.e. 30 seconds, there is no rise in accuracy of the measured result, as the training pulse falls too much over a longer counting time.

Thanks to modern technology it is now possible to take an exact ECG training pulse rate using a cableless pulse rate measuring kit. Each participant then wears a chest-belt (transmitter) and a pulse watch (receiver) where the pulse rate can be seen at any time. With the aid of this piece of equipment, one can dispense with time-consuming and inaccurate manual pulse readings.

A special kind of pulse watch has been developed for aerobics called the cardio-control-system. It is possible with this to transmit the readings of the participants' chest-belt in a larger display onto the wall, so that the aerobics trainer can watch the pulse rate of all her participants during the entire aerobics class.

Alongside the objective criteria of intensity measurement, an important part is also played by the subjective criterion, whereby the participants work out their own optimum training intensity with the aid of the Borg-Scala. This tries to sort out rather more subjective feelings of exertion using the numbers 6-20 (from: very, very light = 7 to: very, very hard = 19). One assumes here that the participants already have some experience of endurance loading and have a feeling for loading intensity and loading levels. This method is not particularly reliable, of course, as a subjective criterion, but it is of value when assessing the overall load.

Together with the objective and subjective criteria of measuring intensity levels, there still remains the most practicable alternative and that is, measuring intensity using someone else, usually the aerobics trainer. External indications of training too intensively are a very red face, a white triangular area around the nose and mouth (shows acute circulatory weakness), too much sweating (with beginners, whose bodies must first learn how to sweat), irritating cough (after training), loss of concentration (reduced ability to concentrate) and shortage of breath.

Controlling Intensity

During the cardio part the aerobics trainer has various ways of controlling exertion at her disposal (i.e. reducing or increasing the level of loading intensity) in order to optimise as much as possible the conditional level of the training unit for her participants. Experienced participants can control their training intensity themselves, using the same principle.

The aerobics trainer can increase the intensity by a choice of steps or movements, raising and lowering the body's centre of gravity, adding high-impact movements, larger radial movements of arms and legs, special movements and faster music or, equally by reducing all of these elements, she can vary the intensity.

The basic principle remains the same, that the aerobics trainer can control the intensity level by her choice of movements, because various patterns of movement vary in their level of exertion (e.g. Jumping Jacks are much harder work than Knee Lifts).

Adding high-impact movements undoubtedly increases the physiological intensity, but it also raises the bio-mechanical stress. Thus, a combination of low- and high-impact elements has proved to be the best way of structuring the cardio part.

We do not recommend additional use of hand or foot weights to increase intensity in the cardio part as there has proved to be a disproportionate rise in injury.

If it looks as if the participants are being conditionally overstretched, then all these "increase options" can be set in reverse.

5.3.4 Aerobic Choreography and Teaching Methods

When talking about aerobic choreography, one means the formal structuring of heart and circulatory training i.e. planning to insert patterns of movement, how they fit into the given time and space and how to combine them. Choreography is not an end in itself, but rather it should facilitate an optimum, efficient, safe and motivating type of training. Planning the choreography demands the trainer's knowledge of certain principles within which she can give her creativity free reign.

Demands of Aerobic Choreography

The choreography must be comprised of patterns of movement which flow into each other harmoniously and contain gentle transfer from one movement to the next, thus avoiding any "stumbling" into the next movement. Thus, it is not a good idea to combine "Biceps Curl" with "Chest Press", or "Push Touch" with "Hopscotch".

The choreography must fit the space available; i.e. high-impact elements cannot be done on a hard, non-springy floor, and a carpeted floor is unsuited to turns, putting unnecessary strain on the joints. Sometimes a small room, or too many participants, prevents spacial movements, or movements which are too complex.

The choreography should be weighed up physiologically, changing from intensive to less intensive patterns of movements, so that the participants remain within their optimum training pulse area.

The choreography should also be bio-mechanically balanced and conform to the safety standards for aerobics. If the movements are varied, this avoids one-sided stress on the joints, for example contradictory movements or positions should be omitted, like overstretched joints or unsupported trunk movements.

In choreographic work a few psychological aspects should be taken into consideration. The combination of steps should tax the participants, but also guarantee a feeling of success and enjoyment, despite their complexity. The decisive element here is the teaching-technique skill of the trainer. The teaching method, cueing, confidence with the music and the trainer's ability to work with mirrors are the most important factors in ensuring a safe passage through the choreography.

Foundation Stones on Aerobic Choreography

The basic elements of choreography are a relatively limited number of basic movements of the arms and legs, which can be varied as follows:

Leverage Length
Many movements e.g. "side-lifting" can be done with a long lever (outstretched arm) or a short lever (bent arm).

Movement Plain
A "kick" can be done forwards, diagonally outwards, to the side or backwards.

Rhythmic Variations
A "Step Touch" can be done at full or half speed. Movements can be syncopated i.e. runing against the beat of the music.

Intensity
Depending on the radius of each movement, it can be more or less intensive. Also many step patterns can be done in a high- or low-impact version.

Unilateral/Bilateral
A movement like "front lift" can be done with one or both arms. A step pattern like Grapevine can only be done to one or both sides (there and back).

Direction
A movement can be done in various directions e.g. "Step Touch" sideways or forwards/backwards. Movements can also be done in varying directions in the room i.e. the participants look forwards, to the side or backwards.

As well as ways of varying the patterns of movement, aerobic choreography can be done "travelling", changing direction or with turns. Step combinations are often set up as "floor patterns" i.e. the travelling routes can be marked out, for example, in the shape of an "L", a square or a triangle.

Movements can be combined in many different ways, for example, a step pattern can be linked with various arm movements, but step patterns alone can be put together in all sorts of ways.

Also the way in which training is organised gives scope for creativity. Together with the classic variation "trainer stands in front of the group", one can also train in a circle or a formation, where two or more groups work against each other.

Methodical Procedures

When trying to put across a choreography, the aerobics trainer can use innumerable different aids. Basically one differentiates between methods which convey well-established combinations of movement (method with structured procedure), and methodical types of procedure for training, which do not have any specific "end product" (freestyle method).

Especially when training beginners, whose co-ordinative abilities are not very well developed, one should leave any complex choreography "blocks" alone and concentrate rather on letting the participants practise patterns of movement without any pressure of having to remember movement combinations. The following procedures fit in well here:

Linear Progression

When changing from one movement to the next, only one element of that movement is altered. So, either the arm movement is changed whilst the leg movement remains the same, or only the leg movement, or only the direction, or the way of doing it (high- or low-impact). When learning new movement patterns, the leg movement is practised before the arm movement. This procedure guarantees beginners simple transfers of movement whilst continuing to train their heart and circulation. This is particularly useful when new movements are to be introduced or variations to be practised. This method also does not overtax the participants' ability to remember, because there are no fixed movement combinations at the end of the session.

Top and Tail

Here only two movements are combined, with no extensive combinations of movement.

1. Practise movement A.
2. Practise movement B.
3. Repeat a few times: A-B-A-B-A-B ...
   (The separate movements A and B can also be kept on for longer.)
4. Practice movement C.
5. Repeat a few times B-C-B-C-B-C ...
   (Movement A is no longer done.)
6. Practise movement D, then C-D-C-D-C-D-etc.

When a new movement is put on the end, an earlier starting movement is omitted.

Zigzag

Here one can combine several movements. This method is closer to the building-up methods for combinations of movements described below, because longer combinations can arise from it. However, it always permits an end and new beginning, when the limit of the participants' concentration has been reached.

1. Practise movement A.
2. Practise movement B.
3. Repeat a few times: A-B-A-B-A-B ...
4. Practise movement C.
5. Repeat A-B-C-B-A-B-C-B-A ...
6. Practise movement D.
7. Repeat A-B-C-D-C-B-A-B-C-D ...

The separate movements are run through here in a snake-like formation.

When dealing with advanced participants, who have already internalised the basic movement patterns, one often works with fixed combinations of movements made out of several individual movements. The combination is built up during the course of a lesson, whereby the building-up process in itself constitutes the heart and circulatory training. The participants get a feeling of achievement from running through a complete combination several times. The use of combinations (compared with "freestyle") ensures a greater range of training. Also the participants can anticipate forthcoming movements and therefore train in a more relaxed way. However, this type of lesson plan demands more from the trainer because the combinations must suit the muscle structure, as well as being built up logically and fluently.

Here are a few ways of building up combinations using methodical procedures:

Add on

1. Practise movement A.
2. Practise movement B.
3. Practise movement A nd B together and repeat.
4. Practise movement C.
5. Practise movement A + B + C together and repeat.
6. Practise movement D.
7. Practise movement A + B + C + D together and repeat.

Similarly, one can start using movements E-H, and then the trainer decides whether A-H are attached or not.

Link (Block Method)

1. Practise movement A.
2. Practise movement B.
3. Practise movement A and B together and repeat a few times.
4. Practise movement C.
5. Practise movement D.
6. Practise movement C and D together and repeat a few times.
7. Practise combination A + B + C + D + together and repeat.

The combination A + B + C + D is the end product which can be run through several times. One can do the same with movements E-H, and then add on A-H again if you wish.

Sometimes problems arise when building up combinations of movement along these lines, because some movements are very complex and need careful methodical explanation. Also movement transfers can be particularly difficult, and in this case a range of methodical aids are available to extend the learning time and facilitate explanations.

Arm Work Comes after Leg Work

If the participants have difficulties in carrying out leg and arm movements at the same time, then the leg movement can be practised first. Then the arm movement is added or maybe practised separately, with a simple leg movement like marching to go with it.

Changing Tempo

If learning one movement is particularly difficult, then it can be practised at half speed to start with. A V-Step would then be done to eight beats rather than four, but doubling the tempo to end with.

Holding Pattern Removal

When learning a combination of movements, "holding" patterns like small knee bends or hops are inserted between the individual movements. Then the holding patterns are removed and the whole programme repeated. The holding patterns give more time for learning a combination and make it easier to transfer from one movement to the next.

Layer (Substitute)

In a simple combination of movements one individual movement is replaced by the next of the same length:
Example:

A: Eight steps walking forwards.
B: Eight steps marching on the spot.
C: Eight steps walking backwards.
D: Eight steps marching on the spot.

After practising the combinations A-D, A and C can be replaced by eight steps of jogging or four of Cha Cha; B and D could be replaced by four Step Touches or two Grapevines etc. The combination thus becomes increasingly complex. The participants can decide for themselves whether they do the complicated or simple variations.

Pyramid/Pyramid Upside Down

During the pyramid, the repeat numbers of a movement are increased bit by bit:

Example:
First one Push Touch right, one Push Touch left, repeat,
then two Push Touches right, two Push Touches left, repeat,
then four Push Touches right, four Push Touches left.

During the inverted pyramid the repeat numbers are slowly reduced to the desired number. This technique gives participants time to learn the movement transfers slowly.

Visual Preview

The participants do a simple holding movement (e.g. Marching, Step Touch, Push Touch or Jogging). Meanwhile, the trainer demonstrates the next complex movement pattern to be worked at. The visual information enables the participants to prepare to change over to the next sequence of movement. Finally the trainer and participants practise the movement together, maybe initially at half speed.

As the holding movement nearly always causes a loss of intensity, this minor aid should not be used too often.

There are many ways of building up combinations of movement and no one technique should be used exclusively. A combination of these methods often leads to a much clearer structure than one method on its own. A bit of experimentation with the introduction of techniques creates a sense of security in their use and the trainer will soon realize which is best for her.

However, with the introduction of all these methods comes the advice: moving forward slowly guarantees learning success on the part of the participants and prevents injury. Trainers should exercise patience and support "slower" participants. Movements which are too complicated, frustrate not only the participants, but damage clear technique and effective training.

5.4 Cooling Down

5.4.1 Main Aims

The aim of this phase is to stabilise the circulation by active recovery. By slowly reducing the loading intensity, the pulse rate is lowered and possible collection of blood in the deeper leg veins prevented. The body's basic temperature is slowly reduced to its starting level and metabolic products of muscular stress from the preceding cardio-phase are got rid of faster from the muscles by continuing moving. As well as fulfilling these physiological objectives, cooling down should also contribute towards mental relaxation and release from the previous tension. The pouring out of hormones, produced in larger amounts during exertion (e.g. adrenalin and noradrenalin) is reduced.

5.4.2 Performance

In order to realise these goals one must find suitable step sequences and movement patterns, which are distinguished by a successive reduction in their movement radius and leverage. The arms should not be raised higher than the shoulder-blades. By the time one reaches the stretching exercises at the end of the cooling down the head should remain above the level of the heart to avoid destabilising the circulation situation, which could lead to a circulatory collapse in certain cases.

In all sorts of ways cooling down is at the opposite pole from warming-up. If the aim of warming-up is to prepare for exertion by raising the body's basic temperature, then the aim of cooling down is to lower it again and set processes in motion, which facilitate recovery from exertion. If we work with increasing loads during warming-up, then this process is reversed during cooling down. Both phases have the speed of the music in common, namely 124-136 bpm. The total duration of cooling down should be about five minutes.

The cooling down phase often demands special skill from the aerobics trainers. Many participants are tired after an exhausting cardio-phase and need special motivation from their trainer to keep moving. At the same time, however, the steps and movement patterns on offer should fulfill the physiological aim of stabilising one's circulation. To help solve this problem, simple low-impact step sequences are available, which possibly repeat a movement sequence from the beginning of the cardio-phase (ensuring that movement radii and leverage are always decreasing). This gives the participants a familiar feeling and creates a motivating atmosphere of rounding off the aerobics class.

Another possibility is the use of step patterns in special styles like funk, Lambada, Salsa, tango or waltz. These styles are well-suited to cooling down on account of their slower tempo, and have a motivating effect in that they are a somewhat different form of expression.

At the end of cooling down, muscles should be stretched which have been stressed during the cardio-phase. These is first and foremost the calf muscles (m. gastronemius, m. soleus) and the muscles right up the back of the legs (ischiocrural muscles). This post-aerobic stretch guards against injury and is done in a standing position with one's head above one's heart.

5.5 Floorwork

5.5.1 Main Aims

When discussing floorwork, one means the sum total of all muscle strength endurance exercises which are done during an aerobics class. That means that floorwork exercises need not take place only on the floor, but they can be done standing up.

Floorwork should be a significant part of each aerobics class, and the aerobics trainer should devote at least 15 minutes to it. Depending on the total length of the training unit, floorwork can be extended to take longer. One can even plan a lesson with floorwork at the centre.

Floorwork music speed is between 112 and 128 bpm.

The aim of floorwork is to improve muscle strength and lasting muscle strength. It is also possible to compensate for muscular imbalance with specific floorwork exercises, and thus improve the body posture of the course participants.

Please note that the floorwork section of an aerobics class is neither geared towards transverse muscle growth nor to getting rid of fat. Contrary to many assumptions it is not possible to burn off fat by floorwork alone!

Muscular Imbalance

Everyday stresses and lack of movement can lead to muscular imbalance. The muscles are tense, which lead in turn to degenerative changes in the joints and spinal column. An improvement in one's posture can be brought about by a specific choice of strengthening exercises for any muscle group inclined to be weaker, and stretching exercises for muscle groups showing signs of contraction. The aim is to produce muscular balance, and to take into consideration one's individual posture. So, putting together the right strengthening and stretching exercises is very complicated. Nevertheless, there are a few types of muscular imbalance which occur frequently:

Muscles inclined to contract	Muscles inclined to weaken
• M. trapezius – upper part (hooded muscle) • M. pectoralis – major part (large chest muscle) • M. erector spinae (low back stretcher) • M. iliopsoas (hip bender) • M. adductor group (leg raiser) • M. ischiocruralis (back upper thigh) • M. gastronemius • M. soleus	• M. rhomboideus (rhomboid muscle) • M. serratus anterior (front sawing muscle) • M. erector spinae – middle section (back stretcher) • M. glutaeus maximus (large bottom muscle) • M. rectus abdominis (stomach muscles) • M. tibialis anterior (front skin muscle)

5.5.2 Scientific Principles for Training

The concept "strength", as far as scientific training is concerned, belongs to conditional abilities and can be defined as the basic ability of a human being to overcome and work against resistance by using muscles, i.e. to stop opposition.

The ability to use strength consists of three different components: fast strength, muscular endurance and maximal strength. By maximal strength one understands the highest possible force that the nerve and muscle system, concentrating as hard as one can, generates during maximum contraction. Muscular endurance is the organism's capacity to get tired during lengthy performances of strength. Fast strength is the ability to carry out movements at high speed with reduced resistance.

Basically, two types of working and forms of muscular contraction are to be seen, neither of which appears regularly in its purest form: i.e. the dynamic (moving) and static (stationary) type of muscle work. During the floorwork of an aerobics class it is mainly the dynamic type of working which is favoured.

If one interprets sports training as a process to stimulate reaction, then the prerequisite for effective, performance-increasing, adaptive signs in the body is that the stimuli are applied correctly. If there is not enough stimulus, the necessary threshold of stimulation is not reached and the body does not adapt itself correctly, so the training remains ineffective. On the other hand, if too much stimulus is provided, and here we are talking about overtraining, then wear and tear occur.

So, the Roux rule applies:
"Slight stimuli are pointless, medium stimuli useful but excess stimuli damaging!"

During sports training one is primarily concerned with a moderate amount of strain. This is dependent on strength of stimulus, range of stimulus, length of stimulus, concentration of stimulus, frequency of stimulus, as well as frequency of training.

Principle of Super-compensation
By super-compensation one means the bio-mechanical and physiological restoration of exhausted energy resources over and above the original level before exertion began. Actually, the phenomenon super-compensation is the body's mechanism to defend itself against overexertion. If one applies such impulses regularly over a longer period of time, the body reacts with increased performance i.e. what we are aiming to achieve in our training.

5.5.3 Performance

The most important working material is force of gravity. The aerobics trainer is constantly looking for training positions which train the chosen muscle against resistance from the force of gravity. For advanced participants force of gravity can be increased by additional apparatus (heavy hands, tubes, physio-bands etc). When using physio-bands or tubes, the exercises are carried out against resistance from the bands.

All movements are done slowly (without jerking) and under control (not too lively). Swinging movements put the joints at too much risk.

All exercises should be done across the full movement radius, so that training is effective and one's muscle flexibility is maintained.

The floorwork exercises should be done in such a way that a concentric strengthening stimulus is always practised on the first beat of a phrase. This "working with the music" is regarded as especially motivating by the participants and thus supports the performance of the exercise.

There are a limited number of training positions, which are harmless from a sports medicine point of view if one executes them correctly. To make floorwork a bit more interesting, rhythmic variations are used.

Let's for example have a look at "Crunch" for strengthening the straight stomach muscles: the aerobics trainer could lead the participants into contracting on the first beat of the bar, then tilting the upper body slightly on the second beat, contracting again on the third beat and sinking down again slightly on the fourth beat (1 = high, 2 = low, 3 = high, 4 = low). That is probably the rhythm to which one trains most often.

A rhythmic variation on this would be to contract during two beats and finally to sink down during two beats (1 = high, 2 = high, 3 = low, 4 = low). This variation is somewhat harder than the basic exercise. A further rhythmic possibility, which is a bit more difficult, is to contract during three beats and only sink down for one (1 = high, 2 = high, 3 = high, 4 = low).

The most difficult rhythmic variation is to contract on the first beat, remain still for "2" and "3" and sink down again on the fourth (1 = high, 2 = hold, 3 = hold, 4 = low).

Other Ways of Increasing Intensity

During floorwork the intensity can be increased considerably by lengthening the leverage, retaining the contraction, using larger movement radii, a greater number of repeats, as well as picking up small hand apparatus like heavy hands, tubes or physio-bands (see 7.2).

5.5.4 Exercise Catalogue of the Most Important Strengthening Exercises

This exercise catalogue gives you a kind of minimum repertoire of potential strengthening exercises and shows you, the aerobics trainer, the most important floorwork exercises. This catalogue does not make any claims to be complete!

M. Pectoralis Major (Large Chest Muscle)

Exercise description:	*Butterfly*
Level of difficulty:	Easy
Starting position:	Lying on the back, the upper arms are put down at one's side with the lower arms bent at right angles.
Performance:	The bent arms are brought in front of the body.

Tip: Advanced people can do the same exercise with
                              long leverage (i.e. the arms are stretched out at
                              the side and then brought in front of the body.

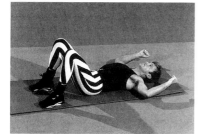 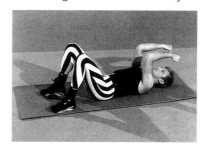

Exercise description: *Press-ups with short leverage*
Level of difficulty: Medium
Starting position: One's body weight rests on the arms, which are
                              fairly wide apart, and the knees. The arms are
                              bent slowly and the body thereby lowered.
Performance: The arms are stretched and the body thus raised again.
Tips: Avoid a hollow back; bottom muscles and tummy
                              should be firmly based to stabilise the lower
                              vertebrae (whole-body tension); do not overstretch
                              the elbow joint.

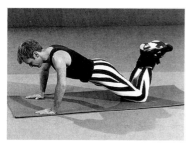 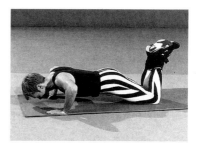

Exercise description: *Press-ups.*
Level of difficulty: Relatively difficult.
Starting position: One's body weight rests on the arms which are
                              relatively wide apart and the tips of the feet.
Performance: See above.
Tips: See above.

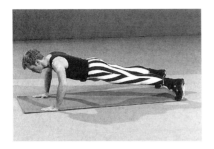 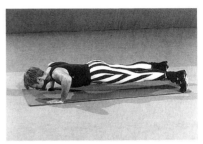

M. Biceps Brachii: (Double-headed Arm-bender)

Exercise description:	*Biceps curl*
Level of difficulty:	Medium
Starting position:	In a standing position, with both feet parallel and arms hanging straight down.
Performance:	The lower arms are bent at the elbow joints, the upper arms keep still.
Tips:	Make use of the movement radius; do not overstretch the elbow joints; wrists remain stable.

Exercise description:	*Biceps curl with hand apparatus (tube)*
Level of difficulty:	Depending on the strength of the tube, relatively difficult.
Starting position:	In a standing position with both feet parallel on the tube, both hands hold a handle of the tube.

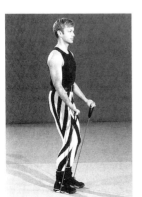 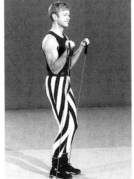

Performance:
The lower arm is bent at the elbow against resistance from the tube.
Tip: Bend and stretch slowly and evenly.

M. Triceps Brachii (Triple-headed Arm-bender)

Exercise description:	*Arm stretching behind one's head*
Level of difficulty:	Easy
Starting position:	In a standing striding position, or sitting down with legs crossed.
Performance:	One arm is stretched upwards and bent behind one's head, which is the starting position, from where the arm is stretched at the elbow joint. The final position is the vertically upright arm.
Tips:	Do not overstretch the arm; keep the upper arm still; shoulders down; do not get a hollow back.

Exercise description:	*Triceps curl with hand apparatus (small dumb-bell in one hand)*
Level of difficulty:	Depends on the weight of the dumb-bell.
Starting position:	In a standing position one hand holds a small dumb-bell, this same upper arm points diagonally backwards, the lower arm is bent.
Performance:	The lower arm is stretched at the elbow.
Tips:	Upper arm remains still! Advanced participants can train both arms simultaneously.

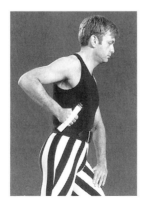 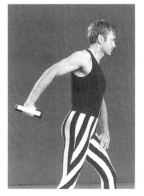

M. Trapezius (Hooded Muscle)
M. Rhomboideus (Rhomboid Muscle)
M. Erector Spinae – Middle Part (Back-stretcher)

Exercise description:	*Arm lifting lying on stomach with short leverage*
Starting position:	Lying on stomach, both arms in a U-position, palms of hands towards the floor.
Level of difficulty:	Medium
Performance:	Both arms are lifted slightly from their U-position and kept there.
Tips:	Upper body stays on the ground; arms should remain in the U-position during the exercise and not wander towards one's bottom; head is in line with the spinal column: avoid a hollow back and no hyper extension of the lumbar vertebrae.

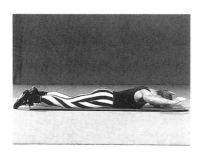

Description of exercise:	*Arm-lifting, lying on one's stomach with long leverage*
Level of difficulty:	Relatively hard

Starting position:

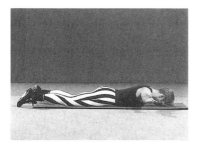

Lying on one's stomach, both arms are stretched out to the side; palms of hands towards the floor.
Performance: Both arms are lifted slightly and kept there.
Tips: See above.

M. Rectus Abdominis (Straight Stomach Muscles)

Description of exercise: *Crunch*

Starting position: Lying on one's back, put down both heels with knees bent (the further the heels are from the body, the harder the exercise).

Level of difficulty: Easy

Performance: Both arms are pulled forward past the sides of the body and at the same time the upper body, including shoulder-blades, is lifted slightly and lowered again, but not completely.

Tips: Keep chin free (there must be enough space for a tennis ball to fit between top part of body and head); look diagonally towards the ceiling without cramping the neck;
head in line with spinal column;
do not pull shoulders forward;
lumbar vertebrae remain fixed to the floor.

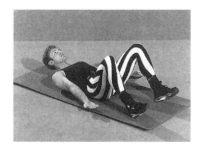 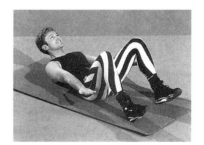

Variations of Arm Position

Exercise description: *Crunch with arms crossed over on one's chest*
Level of difficulty: Easy/medium
Starting position: See above, but both arms are crossed over on one's chest.
Performance: See above.
Tips: See above.

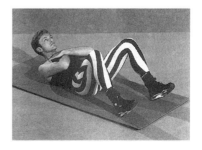

Exercise description:	*Crunch with short leverage*
Level of difficulty:	Medium
Starting position:	See above, but now both arms are crossed behind one's neck.
Performance:	See above.
Tip:	Keep your elbows to the side.

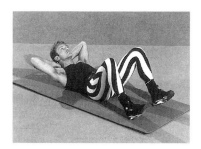

Exercise description:	*Crunch with long leverage*
Level of difficulty:	Difficult
Starting position:	See above, but both arms are folded above the head.
Performance:	See above.
Tip:	This exercise is only suitable for advanced participants.

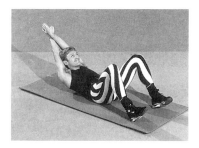

Exercise description:	*Reverse crunch (Pelvic Lift)*
Level of difficulty:	Relatively hard
Starting position:	Lying on one's back, both legs are stretched parallel and upwards with arms under the head.
Performance:	One's bottom is raised slightly and then lowered again by the contraction of the lower stomach muscles.
Tips:	Do not press yourself off the floor with your arms; no leg swinging.

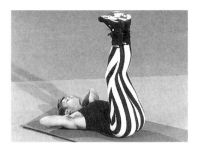 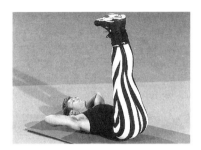

M. Obliquus Externus Abdominis and M. Obliquus Internus Abdominis (Diagonal Stomach Muscles)

Exercise description:	*Diagonal crunch*
Starting position:	See above, but one leg (e.g. the right one) is crossed over the other thigh (outer ankle bone of the right leg is now lying on the left thigh). The arm on the side of the crossed-over leg, in our case the right arm, is stretched out sideways on the ground to stabilise, and the other hand is placed behind the neck.
Performance:	The left shoulder is lifted slowly and diagonally in the direction of the right knee and then lowered again, but not completely.
Tips:	Stabilise the pelvic area well on the ground; no hyper-extension of the pelvic vertebrae area; avoid any swinging of head or arms; do not pull the shoulders forward.

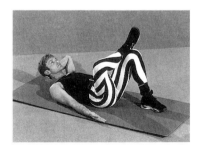 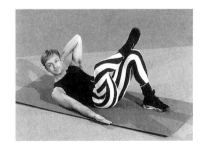

M. Glutaeus Maximus (Large Bottom Muscle)

Exercise description:	*Leg-lifting whilst kneeling (bench position)*
Starting position:	Kneeling and supporting on one's elbows, tense the stomach slightly and keep the back straight. One leg is then stretched out straight backwards and the lower leg bent at right angles, so that the sole of one's foot is parallel with the ceiling. Then the bent leg is lowered to just above the floor.
Level of difficulty:	Medium
Performance:	The bent leg is lifted back to the horizontal and lowered again nearly to the floor, but not put down.
Tips:	Stabilise the pelvic area well to avoid a hollow back; do not turn the pelvis sideways; trunk must not move sideways either; do not lift the leg any higher than horizontal; avoid hyperextension of the neck vertebrae.

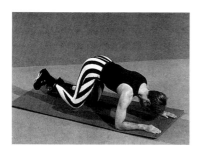 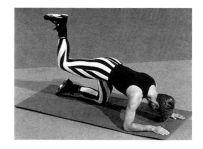

Exercise description:	*Squat (knee bend)*
Level of difficulty:	Hard
Starting position:	Put both legs down a little further apart than the width of your hips; feet are parallel or turned outwards slightly; both hands are supported on the thighs and both legs bent.

Performance:	Both legs are stretched from this starting position and then bent again to a maximum of 90° right angle bend.
Tips:	Do not turn the knee too far; do not push the knee further than the tips of your feet; heels should remain on the ground; do not have too big a radius of movement (knee-bending must not exceed 90°)!

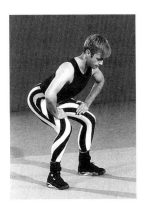 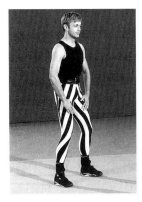

M. Biceps Femoris (Leg-bender)

Exercise description:	*Leg-bending whilst kneeling (bench position)*
Starting position:	Kneeling and supported on both elbows, keep the stomach slightly tense and the back straight. One leg is stretched straight out backwards.
Performance:	The outstretched leg is bent and stretched.
Tips:	Stabilize the pelvic area well to avoid a hollow back; trunk must not slip sideways; move the leg slowly and carefully.

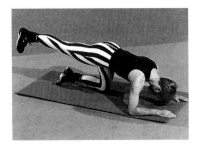 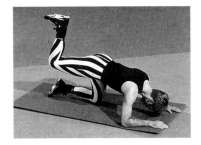

M. Quadriceps (Leg-stretcher)

Exercise description:	*Plié*
Starting position:	With both legs relatively wide apart (this varies from person to person depending on hip width), both tips of feet are turned outwards slightly, with the knees pointing towards them and then bent.
Performance:	Out of the bent position, the legs are stretched and then bent again.
Tips:	The size of the stride must be big enough for the knees to remain over the tips of the feet and not go beyond them; make use of your movement radius, the knee joint can be bent up to 90° but no further; Avoid positioning the knee wrongly; always keep it in the same direction as the tips of your feet.

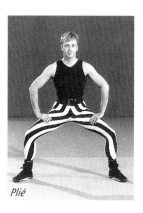

Plié

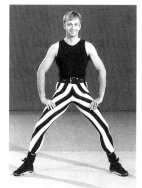

Exercise description:	*Flexed Lunge (striding step – knee bend)*
Starting position:	Both legs are in the basic position for Plié, then the whole body is turned to the side; one knee is bent as for the stretching of the hip-bender and then finally lowered.
Performance:	Both legs are stretched from this starting position and then bent again.
Tips:	Do not overstretch the legs; knee joint of front leg must remain above the ankle; heel of front leg stays on the floor!

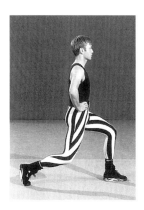 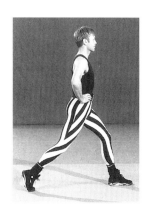

Adductors (Thigh Straightener)

Exercise description:	*Lifting the adductors*
Starting position:	Lying on your side with underneath leg slightly bent to stabilise you, put your lower arm flat on the ground, rest your head on it and put your upper arm for support above your body.
Performance:	The upper leg is lifted and put down again, but not completely.
Tips:	Do not tip your pelvis backwards; do not rotate your upper leg outwards; do not choose too big a movement radius; do the movement slowly and carefully.

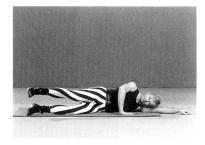 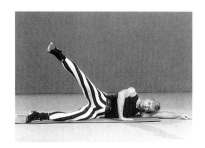

Adductors (Thigh Tightener)

Exercise description: *Lifting the adductors*
Starting position: Lying on your side with the upper leg bent, then brought down again forwards. Put the lower arm flat on the ground, put your head on it and give yourself extra support by putting your upper arm above your head.
Performance: The underneath leg is raised and put down again, but not completely.
Tips: Knee joint and tips of feet point forwards; the leg is raised parallel to the ground; the pelvis should not be tilted upwards.

Lifting the adductors

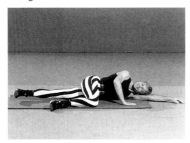 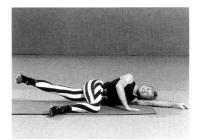

5.6 Stretching

5.6.1 General Aims

The stretching-phase at the end of an aerobics class aims to prevent the contraction of any groups of muscles which were used a lot in the previous exercise phases by now stretching them. In addition to this, one should gain considerable improvement in the flexibility of one's joints. Both of these aspects, avoiding muscle contraction and improving joint flexibility, help prevent injury and improve performance.

5.6.2 Physiological Principles

In between each muscle's muscle fibres are sensors which, due to their springy nature, can be stretched and made longer. These muscle spindles register changes in muscle strength. If the muscle is stretched too fast or too far (i.e.

longer), the muscle spindles then cause the stretched muscle to contract by a reflex arc. This so-called stretching reflex protects the muscle from overstretching and any injuries thus caused (muscle fibre tears).

Sensors are not only to be found in the muscles, but also in the connecting area between muscles and tendons. Working differently from the muscle spindles, these tendon spindles measure mainly the state of tension in the tendons. Tendon spindles (also called "Golgi-organs") have a higher stimulation threshold than the muscle spindles i.e. the tension in the tendons caused by contraction or stretching of the muscles, must be very powerful before the tendon spindles react. Once the threshold is reached, however, the tendon spindles, unlike the muscle spindles, cause the muscles to relax, in order to reduce the tugging on the tendons. This reaction is known as an inverse stretching reflex.

5.6.3 Mobility

A guide for mobility is from the amount of movement radius in any one joint. This movement radius is limited by certain factors:

1. The joint structure
2. Stretchability of the muscle-connecting tissue, the tendons, ligaments and skin
3. One's age
4. One's sex
5. How warm the mobility apparatus is
6. Time of day.

In sports medicine literature, dynamic mobility and static mobility are separate entities. Dynamic mobility describes the largest possible movement radius in a joint, which can be achieved from the contraction of the agonist whilst stretching the opposite antagonist simultaneously. By static mobility, one means the largest possible movement radius, which can be achieved by the antagonist's ability to contract.

5.6.4 Dynamic and Static Stretching

Analogous to dynamic and static mobility, one can differentiate between dynamic and static stretching. Dynamic stretching is active or passive. If active dynamic stretching is being done, the level of stretching in a muscle depends on the level of contraction in its opposites. The speed and radius, at which the stretching position is reached determines whether one can talk about ballistic stretching or range of motion stretching. Ballistic stretching is done quickly and is characterised by rocky or springy movements. This sort of stretching was one of the favourite and most-often-used stretching exercises in the early stages of the aerobics movement. Many other kinds of sport still use it as a central feature of their training programme. Meanwhile, indications show that ballistic stretching is an unsuitable stretching exercise for leisure sportsmen as well as within an aerobics class. Two factors are against ballistic stretching: 1. The rocking movement used in ballistic stretching causes the stretched muscle to be stretched much further than normal as a result of acceleration forces. 2. The rocking movement probably stimulates the stretching reflex, so that the muscle to be stretched contracts and is then stretched against the contraction. Both of these factors can lead to muscle fibre tears especially in untrained muscles. This has led to ballistic stretching becoming a counter-productive type of stretching in aerobics teaching, because it is potentially damaging. However, if the movement in the stretching position is only done within the normal movement radius for about 4 to 5 seconds, then it is regarded as an effective and safe form of dynamic stretching.

During static stretching the stretching position is reached slowly and then held for a longer period of time. Static stretching can be active. An example is when m. quadriceps is stretched: to get to the stretching position the ischiocrural muscles contract concentrically, whilst contracting isometrically during the holding of the stretching position. We call it passive stretching when external forces, like force of gravity or another person, support the stretching position.

Both forms of stretching are so-called tension and relaxing stretching methods, or PNF techniques (proprioceptive neuromuscular facilition). During these very effective stretching methods the muscle to be stretched is first actively tensed and then relaxed. This can be repeated several times. The physiological basis for this stretching method is the inverse stretching reflex. By the isometric contraction the state of tension in the muscles changes and thereby the amount of pulling of the tendons; however, there is no lengthening of the muscles, so that no stretching reflex is set off. As a result of the increased amount of pull on the tendon spindles are stimulated and these release an inverse stretching reflex. This leads to relaxation of the muscle and thus makes static stretching easier. Static stretching is the most frequent form of stretching at the end of an aerobics class, during which the stretching positions of "easy stretch" should be held for 15-30 seconds. During developmental stretch, the stretching position is taken up again and held for another 15-30 seconds whilst gently intensifying the stretching.

5.6.5 Performance

A few practical tips for healthy and efficient stretching:

1. Only stretch after you have warmed up: only warmed-up muscles can be stretched safely and efficiently.
2. Only go so far in the stretching position, until you feel a slight pulling in the muscle area you wish to stretch. Avoid pain at all costs. If the muscle starts to shake, then it is being overstretched.
3. Breath quickly and evenly when stretching, because this increases the relaxation effect. Help your muscles to stretch by relaxing mentally yourself.
4. Take up a comfortable position for stretching, because you cannot relax properly if uncomfortable.
5. Hold a stretching position for 15-30 seconds.

In the following survey the most important stretching positions at the end of an aerobics class are introduced:

1. Stretching the m. gastronemius (see p. 89).
2. Stretching the ischiocrural muscle group (see p. 89).
3. Stretching the ischiocrural muscle group.
4. Stretching the ischiocrural muscle group.

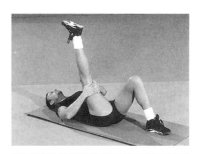

Performance: Leave head, collar bone and lower back in contact with the floor. Grab your calf or thigh and pull your leg towards you slowly.

Tip: Greater flexibility is needed to stretch the lower leg.

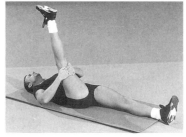

5. Stretching the m. quadriceps.

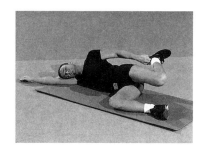

Performance: Head is placed on the upper arm, stomach and bottom muscles tensed tightly; with the same side of the body's hand grab your foot and pull it carefully towards your bottom.

Tip: For some participants it is more comfortable to grab hold of the shoe.

6. Stretching the m. erector spinae and m. gluteus max.

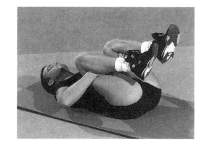

Performance: head and shoulder-blades lie close to the floor; embrace the thighs with the arms and pull the thighs slowly towards the body.

Tip: Make sure you leave head and shoulder-blades relaxed on the floor.

7. Stretching the m. pectoralis major.

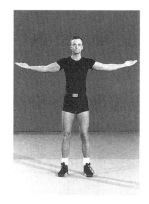

Performance: Body posture in basic position with arms stretched out backwards. If the palms of the hands point upwards, this intensifies the stretching.

Tip: Avoid a hollow back (contraction of stomach muscles). This exercise can be done sitting down.

8. Stretching the m. triceps brachii.

Performance: Body posture in basic position, then pull the elbow carefully behind your head with your free hand.

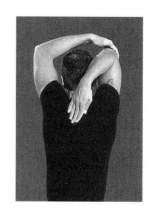

Tip: Avoid a hollow back (contraction of stomach muscles) and relax the back of your neck. This exercise can also be done sitting down.

9. Stretching the adductors.
Performance: Sit firmly on the ground with collar bone above hips. Grab hold of your ankles and tilt your upper body forwards slightly.

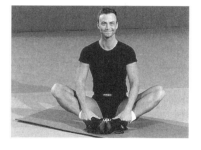

Tip: Avoid a rounded back (pull your shoulders back), and do not over-stretch the neck.

A further aim of the stretching phase is to give the participants a feeling of relaxation at the end of an aerobics class and so enhance their feeling of well-being. In order to stretch efficiently and safely and to create a relaxed atmosphere, a few other external factors must be considered:

1. Room temperature: stretching and relaxing only make sense if the room temperature is high enough for the participants not to freeze when they take up their stretching positions. As they will have all sweated by the end of an aerobics class, it is advisable that we recommend their putting some extra clothing on.

2. Music: the music should support a relaxing atmosphere and have virtually no recognisable text. Instrumental pieces are best for this, because sung or spoken texts take concentration away from the stretching and can make it difficult to hear the trainer's instructions.

3. Instructions: the aerobics trainer should try to speak quietly and calmly but also clearly. By modulating her voice, the trainer can create a pleasant and relaxing atmosphere, which supports the participants' stretching.

Sometimes one can add some deep relaxation to the stretching-phase. This is a good time to do it, as the participants are well-prepared for further relaxation by the previous stretching. There are a number of possible relaxation methods i.e. relaxation through self-hypnosis, progressive muscle relaxation, religious meditation, transcendental meditation, yoga, hypnosis, functional-relaxation and the bio-feedback method. When finishing an aerobics class with relaxation, elements from progressive muscle relaxation and relaxation through self-hypnosis have proved useful. We are not able to give a complete survey about these relaxation methods within the bounds of this book.

6. Do's and Don'ts – Counter-productive Exercises

Every aerobics teacher should constantly review her repertoire, keeping the aim "aerobics as a healthy sport" in mind. Many exercises where one hopes for a certain kind of effect from training are either not functional or can be done incorrectly. They can even present a health risk and lead to injury if done for too long or too intensely.

An aerobics trainer should always have a good knowledge of anatomy and physiology and, above all, keep up-to-date with research. This is the main requirement for being able to select functional exercises to teach, which take the findings of sports science into consideration.

There is undoubtedly a wide variety of counter-productive exercises, but we will only cover the most important non-functional exercises here:

The following exercises should be removed from your exercise catalogue:

1. "Bending the trunk sideways"
Intended effect: Stretching the m. latissimus dorsi.

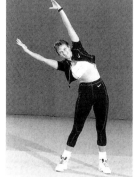

Don't: Bend the trunk sideways without support.
Danger: Wrong strain on the intervertebral discs, overstretching the longitudinal ligament and the small vertebral joints. Possibility of trapped nerves by reducing the size of the spinal channel.

Do: Support one hand on the thigh, hip remains steady, legs slightly bent, bottom slightly tensed, head in neutral position and the other arm pulled diagonally towards the ceiling.

2. "Trunk bending forwards"
Intended effect: Stretching the m. erector spinae.

Don'ts: Bend the trunk forward without support.
Danger: Incorrect strain on the intervertebral discs, greater pressure on the disc around L4/ L5.

Do: See "Warming-up", stretching the m. erector spinae.

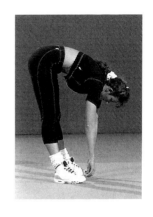

3. "Windmill"
Don't: Tense and stretch the vertebral column at the same time. Too much strain on the discs L4/ L5 in the pelvic area at its weakest point. Damage to the intervertebral discs. No functional exercise for stretching.

Do: See "Warming-up", stretching for the m. erector spinae.

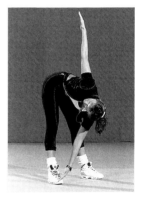

4. "Head circling"
Intended effect: Stretching the m. trapezius.

Don't: Circle your head in a complete circle. By overstretching the neck vertebrae backwards, the vertebral joints and vertebral artery could be damaged and cause dizziness.

Do: Half circles over the chest-bone to the right and left shoulder, and then back at a slower tempo.

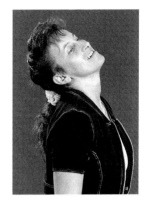

5. "Plough"
Intended effect: Stretching for the back muscles.

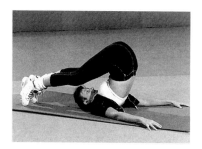

Don't: Do too much overstretching of the rear longitudinal ligament in the spinal column, which brings about unphysiological pressure on the intervertebral discs ("squashing"). One's whole body weight rests on the neck vertebrae.

Do: See "Warming-up", stretching for m. erector spinae.

6. "Knee bend"
Intended effect: Strengthening the leg muscles.

Don't: Bend the knee more than 90° at its joint. The muscular apparatus is no longer used actively, the load is put on the ligaments and cartilage in the knee joint. The thigh bone (femur) presses against the knee-cap (patella).

Do: No knee bends deeper than 90°. The knees point towards the toes, which are turned outwards slightly, with one's weight on the heels.

7. "Sit-ups" – stomach-muscle strengthening.

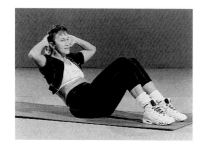

Don't: During sit-ups it is mainly the hip-bender (m. ileopsoas) which is trained; if m. ileopsoas is pulled too much affecting the lumbar vertebrae, additional back problems can arise.

Do: See under "Floorwork", strength-ening of the m. rectus abdominis – "Crunches".

8. "Scissor-legs and double leg lifts"
Intended effect: Stomach muscle exercise.

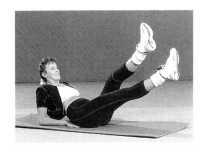

Don't: The turning point is in the hip joint. A greater lumbar vertebral lordosis is caused by the heavy weight of the legs, m. iliopsoas also pulls on the lumbar vertebrae, so that the vertebral discs can be damaged by compression if the exercise is done for too long.

Do: See under "Floorwork", strengthening of m. rectus abdominis, "Reverse Crunch".

9. "Cobra"
Intended effect: Stomach muscle stretching.

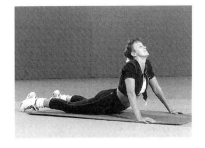

Don't: Stretch the spinal column too far (hyperstretching), or you will damage the little vertebral joints and the intervertebral discs. The spinal column can be jolted especially around the lumbar vertebrae.

Do: Stomach-muscle stretching is unnecessary for most people as these muscles are more inclined to be too weak rather than too short. One could possibly do some brief relaxation lying on one's back with arms and legs outstretched and stomach muscle slightly tensed (reduces too much lumbar lordosis).

10. Strengthening the back-stretcher (m. erector spinae) by overstretching (hyperextension)

Don't: Causes damage to the lumbar vertebrae especially around L4 (lumbar vertebrae) and S1 (sacrum), intensifying an already-existing hyperlordosis.

Do: Lying on your stomach, keep arms outstretched alongside the head and as an extension of the trunk. Point your fingertips towards the ceiling ("Heel shove"). Arms and legs lifted slightly off the ground (increase tension) with head remaining in line with the spinal column. (Instruction: "Someone is pulling you apart.") The back muscles are strengthened by this exercise and the spinal column stretched.

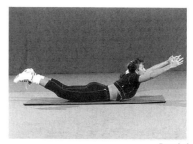

Don´t!

11. "Dog at tree"
Intended effect: Strengthening the bottom muscles.

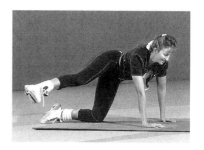

Don't: No strengthening of the large bottom muscle, rather than an overloading of the smaller outer hip-rotators. Damage to the lumbar vertebrae – sacrum area because of the pelvic girdle's evasive movement to the side.

Do: See under "Floorwork", strengthening the m. glutaeus maximus.

12. Strengthening the abductor group with supported lower arm.

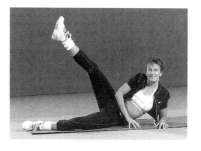

Don't: Considerable distortion of the vertebral column can be caused by the supported lower arm and outward-turned hip. The intervertebral discs are squashed and the smaller vertebral joints are damaged.

Do: See under "Floorwork", strengthening the adductors.

13. "Hurdle sitting"
Intended effect:
Stretching the ischiocrural group.

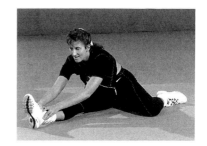

Don't: Damage to the ligaments due to turning and compressing the cartilage in the bent knee.

Do: See under "Stretching", stretching the ischiocrural group.

7 Variations

7.1 Interval Training

The interval method is a general term for a type of training with systematic alternation of physical exertion and recovery phases (changing from high-intensity exercises to phases of a less intense nature).

One differentiates between extensive and intensive interval training.
The extensive interval method is characterised by a large volume and relatively little intensity. The main objective is to improve one's aerobic capacity.
The intensive interval method, on the other hand, is characterised by a smaller volume but higher intensity, where one aims to improve the anaerobic potential.

Sports science divides interval methods into groups depending on their individual exertion duration:

• Short-time-interval: length of loading and recovery phase between 15 seconds and a minute.
• Medium-time-interval: length of interval between one minute and eight minutes.
• Long-time-interval: length of interval between eight and 15 minutes.

The principle of the "reward" break means that there is no complete recovery to come. The recovery phases are structured actively i.e. with the pulse rate at about 120 bpm.

The advantages of interval training are an improvement in the combustion of carbon dioxide, the anaerobic and aerobic capacity respectively as well as improved oxygen absorption. As a result of the active regeneration in the recovery phase, the accumulated lactic acid in a tired muscle can be got rid of more quickly.
A psychological advantage of this sort of interval training is that the participants reach their outermost limit, knowing that a recovery phase follows.

Examples of various recovery and loading ratios:

1. Loading phase = 1 minute/recovery phase = 3 minutes (medium-time-interval). This is where the pulse rate in the loading phase is the same or higher than 85% of the maximum heart beat rate.
2. Loading and recovery phase last the same length of time e.g. 1 minute strain and 1 minute recovery, or 2 minutes strain and 2 minutes recovery. Intervals of the same length are possible during a short-time-interval or a long-time-interval. When setting up a course, it is better to use longer interval phases of 1-5 minutes.

Examples for interval training in the area of aerobics:

Loading phase	Duration	Recovery phase	Duration
Skippings or sprints	1 min.	March or Step Touch	3 mins.
High-impact aerobics	3 mins.	Muscle strengthening	1 min.
Step Power Moves	2 mins.	Muscle strengthening	2 mins.
High-/low-impact Aerobics	3 mins.	Step-aerobics	3 mins.
Slide training	4 mins.	Step-aerobics	3 mins.

The range of possibilities has plenty of scope for more.

To prevent the pulse rate dropping too low, one should work with the large muscle groups in the muscle-strengthening section. Knee-bending and striding steps are well-suited to this, and small dumbells can also be included in upper body work.

Examples of a 60-minute course unit:
• Warm-up: 10-15 minutes
• Interval training: 25-30 minutes, ratio of loading to recovery phase 3:1 (seven intervals). If muscle-strengthening exercises are done in the recovery phase, please note the recommended speed. (about 112-128 bpm). Specially-produced music cassettes have appeared on the market to use here.

- Cool-down: 3 to 5 minutes.
- Floorwork: Maybe five stomach muscle exercises for 5-10 minutes.
- Stretching: at least five minutes.

By using interval variations, lesson illustrations can be varied and interesting, so that there is no danger of boredom and the participants continue to be challenged afresh.

7.2 Additional Apparatus

Within the framework of muscle strengthening, various additional pieces of apparatus can be used in the floorwork part of an aerobics class, which increase the range of effective and safe strengthening exercises. Also the intensity of stimulus for strengthening exercises is increased.

The range of extra apparatus is being extended all the time, but not all these aids can be universally used, some have very limited usage. The following pieces of apparatus can be used in different ways and have already established themselves on the open market.

"Heavy hands" are small additional weights which, due to the way they are constructed, can be held in the hands safely and comfortably for quite a long time. They are used for strengthening the upper body muscles, and are offered at various weight levels.

"Weight-cuffs" are usually fixed around the ankles with Velcro, and help to strengthen leg and bottom muscles. They are also available at different weight levels.

"Body bar" is a long-dumb-bell-rod (without weight discs) also available in lighter and heavier versions.

Elastic bands are available in all sorts of shapes and sizes – in open or ring format, in various lengths and strengths and also with handles. They are called exertube, exerring, rubberband, physio band, physio tape etc. They can be used across the whole range of strengthening exercises.

7.2.1 Use of Additional Apparatus

The use of additional apparatus for strengthening exercises puts extra demands on the participants and trainers alike. For the participants, their use means greater co-ordinative and conditioning strain than in an exercise without such apparatus. The apparatus must be used and mastered safely over and above safe and accurate movement and body posture. Inadequate stabilising of the trunk and joints, and poor movement control, can put wrong loads on spinal column, joints and muscles.

Greater resistance is given to a movement by strengthening the force of gravity or from the tugging or the elastic bands. Therefore, by using additional apparatus as opposed to an exercise without them, training acquires a more powerful stimulus.

Consequently, additional apparatus should not be used when training beginners, but only when exact sequences of movement to be performed have become automatic, and the intensity of training does not overstretch the participants.

The trainer needs to have a deeper understanding of anatomical-physiological factors when using additional apparatus. Also, she must pay closer attention to how the participants are doing an exercise and correct any wrong movements.

Additional apparatus is used almost exclusively in the floorwork part of an aerobics class. In the cardio-phase one should not be working with elastic bands or with weight-cuffs. Heavy hands can sometimes be used if the leg work is not too complicated (keep it simple with low-impact movements), a moderate music tempo is selected (130 bpm) and arm movements with long leverage are only done at half speed ("New Body" concept of lessons).

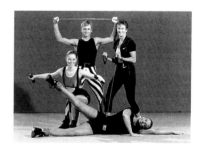

7.2.2 Tips for the Safe and Effective Use of Additional Apparatus

Heavy Hands/Weight-cuffs/Body Bar

- Movements are done slowly and carefully, avoiding any swinging movements.
- Joints are never overstretched.
- If the participants show obvious signs of tiredness from training with additional weights, then train further but without weights.

- Exercises should be so planned that the strengthening stimulus follows naturally out of the movement against the force of gravity.
- During the loading-phase one breathes out.

Elastic Bands

- Before starting training, all bands used should be checked for tears or damage to the handles.
- Each participant should select the correct resistance for her training level.
- The movements are done slowly and carefully without overstretching the joints.
- The band is kept stretched throughout the entire exercise.
- Exercise should be so planned that the band cannot possibly slip from its desired position.
- One should pay attention to correct body posture as well as a neutral position for the wrists.
- In exercises, where one foot or both feet are on the band, one should reduce the tension of the band slowly at the end of the exercise, after which the feet can be removed from it.
- The bands are never held in front of one's own face or that of any other participant.
- Be especially careful when working in pairs.

8 Special Target Groups

8.1 Children and Young People

Many children and young people today move far to little. They sit in school and at their homework. Also in their leisure time they sit predominantly in front of the television, watch videos and play at the computer, all activities, which are mainly done sitting down. The increasing amount of traffic on the roads, increasing violence and growing misuse of drugs, means that parents can no longer let their children play unsupervised in the road. This, subsequently, has led to lack of movement being a universal phenomenon even in children and young people, which carries a considerable health risk, and has a negative influence on all children's development. The urgency for some kind of further preventative measures are indicated by recent statistics:

- 50 to 65%   weak posture
- 30 to 40%   poor co-ordination
- more than 30%   overweight
- 20 to 25%   heart and circulatory weakness or weakness in circulation control (endurance weakness)

Aerobic Sport for Children and Young People as a Form of Compensation

Children's aerobics and teenie-aerobics are trying to respond to this socially-dictated lack of movement and its consequences by offering special movement programmes to children and young people.

The health-promoting effect of aerobics should do children good, especially in the areas of improving their overall endurance performance ability, training their coordinative ability and developing their sense of rhythm.

The principle aim of aerobics with children and young people is the development of a lasting interest in health-promoting movement training. Through a combination of movement, rhythm, music, fun and enjoyment of life the total well-being of children and young people can be improved. Aerobics does something for oneself and one's body and thus acquires a positive feeling towards one's body.

However, before any trainer offers aerobics to children, she should study and understand the following statement:

"The child is not a mini-adult, and its mentality is not only quantitively, but also qualitatively different from that of an adult. This means that a child is not only smaller, but also different."

(*Claparède 1937, quoted by J. Weineck, 1990 p. 51*).

So it would be wrong to simply transfer adult aerobics onto children, as certain physiological and psychological differences must be observed. The amount of training is important when doing aerobics with children, which must be adapted to the age and level of development (biological maturity) and the degree of training they can cope with.

So, here is a sensible way of dividing up the age-groups:

AGE IN YEARS	DESCRIPTION OF TRAINING PROGRAMME
Up to 6	A dance-type of early training (actually has little to do with aerobics)
6 – 10/12	Children's aerobics (simple high-low-impact choreographics and step-aerobics.
10/12 – 14/16	Teen-aerobics (Funk-aerobics or Hip Hop)
after puberty	One would like to see an integration of young people into the usual forms of aerobics (high-low-aerobics, step-aerobics, Funk-aerobics).

Of course, one cannot give exact ages, because the decisive factor is not so much the biological age as biological maturity. It depends on the level of development of children and young people, whether one 12-year-old child copes better with children's aerobics, whereas another might be better placed with the teenies. If it could be organised, it would be a good idea to subdivide children's aerobics groups still further.

Motivational aspects still play a big role when working with children. Children's aerobics must be full of variety, last a relatively short time and be suited to them, so that it is enjoyable, stimulates their imagination and can be done intensively.

Once an interest in aerobics has been roused, then maintaining that motivation should not be difficult, if you take note of the following tips. How you carry out your classes determines whether the Children enjoy aerobics or not and also whether the training programme is successful.

Special Features in Training Children and Young People

According to scientific evidence there is little point in doing general endurance training (mainly aerobics) with children until they are at Junior School (6-10 years). But once they have reached this age, the aerobic exercises should be done at least twice a week for at least 15 minutes at a time, in order to have the desired positive effect on the heart and circulatory system.

Please note that children have a higher pulse rate. Junior School Children have a stress pulse rate of 170 bpm, which is no cause for alarm. Observe carefully that none of the children gets a "white mouth-nose-triangle" during training.

As the mechanism for regulating one's temperature is not as well-developed in children as in adults, children can overheat more easily, so ensure that enough liquid is available to compensate for this.

Also, looked from a scientific training point of view, there are no objections here to dynamic strength training with suitable stimuli. However, the aerobic trainer must realise that pre-pubertal children can indeed increase the strength potential of their muscles, but not any transverse muscle increase (hypertrophy).

Practical Tips and Incentives for Children's Aerobics

- Please note that children's aerobics is group training without any competitive character or sense of contest. Show the children how they can enjoy getting into shape and stay that way.
- Music with a 4/4 beat is needed for children's aerobics. Please choose music that appeals to the children or let them bring their own music. Children are very well-motivated if they can provide their own cassettes. If a child brings suitable music, do not fail to use it.
- Children can only concentrate for short periods of time. On the one hand, children should learn in their aerobics to work carefully through a particular choreography, but do not overdo it. If you see that the children cannot concentrate any more, introduce a little game, (catching for example) to relax them. You only need to ask the children for a few game ideas and you will have a variety to choose from.

- Set up your children's aerobic choreographies in an imaginative but easy way, so that all the children can do them easily. Make room for "little choreographies" as well within your programme.
- Do not be afraid of repeats, because children need time to internalise their newly-learnt movements.
- Finish each lesson with a mini-choreography, which is counted to a song and forms the sum-total of the lesson. If you have difficulties in putting across your planned choreography, then screen the point you have reached with the song.
- Give your children's aerobics choreographies the sense of a "show", so that each choreography has a beginning and a closing scene.
- Try to organise little "performances".
- Respect the children as children and do not treat them as mini-adults.

Teen-aerobics

The young people's, or teenage stage, is a very sensitive one where various processes are taking place i.e. maturing, finding one's identity, development of one's own values and ideas, detaching oneself from the family, desire for independence and the search for a meaningful use of one's leisure time, as they change from being a child to being an adult.

It is well-known that lots of young people stop any sporting activity at this stage of their lives, and once they have decided on an "inactive" life, it is very difficult to interest them in sport and movement; however, there are at the moment other types of sports to rouse their enthusiasm. One just needs to find the right starting point. The basic need for sport must be re-awakened, and the opportunity for this is already there, because young people are, by nature, full of a sense of movement. Lack of movement is merely a result of wrong development within our society.

Re-activating one's natural need to move in an up-to-date way, seems to have been successful through commercial offers from the world of "fashionable" sport, backed up by expensive advertising. This means that traditional basketball is "out" but streetball with all the appropriate equipment is "in". Similarly with roller-skating, where traditional roller-skating is "out" but roller-blading is "in". Probably one can say the same about aerobics i.e. that traditional gymnastics is "out", but high-, low-, step- and Funk-aerobics are "in".

To try and rouse enthusiasm amongst young people for sport and movement, teen-aerobics has adopted another trend from America (Hip-

Hop-culture meets cardio-fitness) and then created lesson scenes like "Funky kids" or "MTV Moves". As indicated by the lesson headings, they contain a special type of aerobics, which have made names for themselves or the aerobic scene with "Funk-aerobics", "Funky", "Hip-Hop", or "Street-Jam".

8.2 Pregnant Women

About ten years ago, in 1985, the American College of Obstetricians and Gynecologists (ACOG) laid down guidelines for sports training for pregnant women, based on research at the time and saying that each pregnant woman should be given the opportunity to do sport safely herself and for her unborn child. Meanwhile, more recent research has set some of these earlier strict recommendations in a different light.

Two of the most important problems, when discussing endurance sport in pregnancy, are the consequences of the mother's overheating and her blood distribution during any physical activity.

Overheating

The serious consequences of raising the mother's basic body temperature are deformities in the unborn child. So far, this has only been proved conclusively in animal experiments. Whether, and to what extent similar effects are apparent in human beings has not yet been scientifically proved. But, one can say with certainty that endurance training done at a lower than maximum level (about 65% VO_2 max.) only causes the mother's temperature to rise to a moderate level which is below the critical level for the unborn child. A woman who has been in training before she became pregnant, will be in a better position to control her rise in temperature by more sweating, so that the foetus does not come to any harm. Women with no complications during pregnancy, who have trained regularly before they became pregnant, can carry on with their aerobic training without any danger, provided that they train at a lower level.

Blood Distribution

Sporting activity leads to blood distribution away from the central organs into the muscles used. This normally sensible process could, in pregnant women, lead to the placenta's receiving less blood and therefore the foetus receiving less oxygen and nourishment than it needs, if the mother is doing sport. This thought has caused the ACOG to recommend that pregnant women should only train for 15 minutes at a time and at low intensity. This recommendation also applies to untrained women.

The results of recent studies also indicate that aerobic training in previously trained pregnant women can have positive effects: i.e. in the early stages of pregnancy aerobic training leads to relatively greater growth in the placenta than in pregnant women who do not continue their endurance training. In the final term of pregnancy, aerobic training can increase the functional capacity of the placenta by around 30% and thus give the unborn child a better blood supply.

Further Changes during Pregnancy

The hormone "relaxin" is produced from the fourth month onwards. During the course of the pregnancy this hormone leads to changes in the connecting tissues and relaxes ligaments and tendons in the pelvic area to make it easier to give birth in due course. Other joints are similarly destabilised and so there is a danger of damaging them during stretching exercises.

Practical Tips

In conclusion, one can say that pregnant women who have already trained regularly before becoming pregnant, and who are enjoying pregnancy without complications, can continue training but must note certain restrictions i.e. that the aim of training is to maintain but not increase their fitness. For the untrained but pregnant, pregnancy is not the time to start a sportive training programme.

Aerobics during pregnancy can contribute to the mother's and unborn child's general well-being. If you observe the following points, you will help expectant mothers to take part in your course safely and successfully:

• The pregnant woman should train regularly (2 to 3 times/week).
• The training pulse should not be more than 140 bpm.
• From the start of the fourth month exercises on one's back should not be done for longer than two minutes.
• Knee-bending should not exceed a 45° angle.
• Extreme stretching of the adductors should be avoided.
• Bending the upper body forwards should never be done unsupported.
• The pregnant woman should not use any additional weights, and should not do any fast rotational movements.

- For safety reasons one should avoid high-impact step patterns.
- It is proved advisable to give a pregnant woman a place in the front row, so that she can always be monitored. However, because some exercises can only be done in a modified form, it is a good idea to let her have a place at the side.

Over and above all of these points comes a doctor's verdict: sporting activity including participation in an aerobics class is only allowed if the doctor sees no objection to continuing training during pregnancy.

8.3 Older People

The age structure of western industrial society is developing more and more from an "age pyramid" (lots of young people at the base and less and less older people, the higher the age rises) in the direction of an "age mushroom" (less young people at the base, lots of people in the higher age groups). In 1989 almost 13% of the total population was older than 65. These figures indicate a ten-fold increase of the older population since 1900. Between 2010 and 2030, when the birth explosion years reach old age, this number is expected to rise again. So, in the future, we will be dealing with more and more older participants (ourselves included).

The group of older people includes the 60-100 year-olds, that is at least four decades, but we cannot look at them all together, in the same way that we cannot talk about all 10-50 year-olds or 20-60 year-olds in the same breath. The old people are a heterogenous group by themselves. Modern differentiations like "the young old people" or "the old old people" (to which group, unkindly, the over 80's belong) do not help either, especially since as one gets older, the number of years tells you less and less about one´s mental and physical state, one's physical well-being, about abilities and achievements or types of experience and behaviour. The chronological age is separated from the "functional age", so that we may as well meet "old old people" in 55 year-olds or "young old people" in 85 year-olds. The Americans are trying to make clear the expression "functional age", by talking about the "go go's", the "slow go's" and the "no go's"!

So that as many elderly people as possible belong to the "go go's", physical activity plays a vital role. Many studies have proved that older people who do endurance sport suffer much less from degenerative and chronic diseases of the joints (arthritis, arthrosis), of the bone (osteoporosis), of their heart and circulatory system (high blood pressure, coronary heart disease) or other systemic diseases (e.g. diabetes mellitus), than their inactive contemporaries. But it is also important in old age to improve one's muscle power and endurance muscle strength. Strong muscles guarantee better body posture and help prevent many of the accidents occuring often in old age by falling over. Particularly in later periods of life, which are affected by impaired ability to function physically and mentally any more, physical activity makes a decided improvement on one's quality of life.

Therefore, it is high time to make aerobics accessible to the aged as well. This is especially important because the aerobics movement has had a predominantly youthful image for a long time. Aerobics training maintains so many factors important to one's general health e.g. endurance performance potential, oxygen absorption capacity, motor coordination ability, muscle power, endurance muscle strength and flexibility. It is important to note that all these factors are subject to a biological degenerative process as one gets older, if they are not trained consistently. Even if one has not trained for many years, by starting an appropriate aerobics programme, one can aim at improving these factors so important to one's health.

Aerobics Programme for the Elderly?

When planning an aerobics class for the elderly, the following points should be considered:

- With advancing years, joint mobility decreases. This has the greatest effect on the length of warming-up time, which should be longer than in courses for younger people. The exercises for joint-isolation in warming-up should be done especially carefully (and repeated slowly and more frequently).
- As many older people have difficulties in understanding and getting into unaccustomed body positions, all exercises should be especially carefully demonstrated.
- During the cardio-phase, one should train at a lower stress intensity, because older people have much less endurance capability than younger people.
- When setting up step choreographies, one should ensure that the elderly often do not trust their own motor skills and get discouraged more quickly than the young. So, offer simple combinations of steps, which you can make more demanding as the weeks go by.

- Be aware in your choice of music that you are teaching older people who probably have little or no experience of the latest pop music trends. In spite of this you should choose music which motivates you personally, and you could compromise with a colourful mixture of various music genres. Apart from the style of music, your choice of music should have recognisable "beat", so that all the participants can work in time to the music. The speed of the music should be slower than what you would choose for a younger group, due to the lower performance potential of your elderly participants.
- As chronic diseases are more likely to occur in a group of older participants than in a younger group, you should be informed about the availability of emergency medical treatment. Also very important, when doing aerobics with older people, is to check external conditions like room temperature, state of the floor, where the training is to take place, and the availability of drinks.

In recent decades it is not only the number of older people which has increased, but also living conditions, state of health and the performance potential of this sector of the population which has radically changed. Most of the over 60's can look after themselves, have a good standard of health, manage without any external support, and react flexibly to new demands put upon them. However, public opinion still has a somewhat negative attitude to getting old. The results of scientific investigations prove, however, that the negative consequences of getting older – illness, loneliness and the need to be looked after, are not forced upon us, but rather are due to faulty integration of the elderly into our society. Aerobics can make a contribution towards older people making more contact again with their contemporaries and then regain confidence in their physical performance potential.

8.4 Men

If you have a look round aerobics groups in sports clubs or fitness studios, you will see that until now it is mainly women who have opted to do aerobics courses. The membership statistics of various clubs or studios show, irrespective of where it is, that the male participation in aerobics courses is only about 5-10%. Observations from time to time by aerobics trainers confirm the low attendance of men.

Have men not yet really discovered aerobics? Or are there other reasons why men hesitate to make their way onto an aerobics course?

Surveys amongst men frequently produce comments like "aerobics is too much dancing for men" or "aerobics is not proper sport", "a lot of jumping around", "it requires too much coordination and I cannot manage that". But we must point out that these sort of remarks come from men who have never even tried such a course! These opinions are very widespread amongst men, but are seldom based on personal experience, and tend to reflect an image of aerobic sport which has its historical imprint. For example the first videos available on the market for aerobics depicted almost exclusively women. Women were the target group of market strategists who wanted to sell their product to women. Thus all the advertising slogans were correspondingly directed towards the female sex and, just as in the cosmetics industry, emphasised attractive appearance, youthfulness and physical presence.

In the two intervening decades aerobics has changed drastically. Whereas in the first aerobics programmes, exercises were still shown, which were not only ineffective, but also questionable from a sports medicine point of view, in the meantime, aerobics has developed into an endurance sport which, when done correctly, fulfills all the demands of a healthy, popular sport. Public perception tends to lag behind this development. More recent trends, like Interval Training with Steps or Box-Aerobics, emphasise the strength and achievement aspects of an aerobics class and should therefore obviously include the male market. Whichever motives are in the forefront of these new developments, be they for marketing or health-political reasons, is really of no consequence: what really matters is that we can embrace any development which causes more people to practise some kind of healthy group sport (and this means all age-groups, irrespective of sex stereotypes).

Aerobics can be in dance form, powerful, performance-orientated or playful. Last but not least, it is the personality of the aerobics trainer which gives an aerobic class its character. At the moment, there are more female than male trainers. Statistics from Great Britain for 1994 show that 91% of trainers were women with only 9% men. Corresponding figures for Germany have not been published as yet, but should be comparable. In this same gross imbalance are also the figures on the participants side. If more men decided to get an aerobics trainer licence and teach aerobics, this could make a major contribution to make the activity popular for the male population.

9 Psychological Principles of Aerobics Teaching

In chapter 2 we saw that endurance training, when done regularly, promotes one's physical and mental well-being in a variety of ways. Aerobics is different from other endurance sports in the following areas:

- Greater effectivity:

  More than 1/6 of the total muscle structure is used during an aerobics class, especially the big groups of muscles. This permits a greater degree of dynamic muscle work before tiredness sets in, compared with other types of training. So, one can train for longer and more intensively.

- Preventing injury:

  Frequent repeats of the same movement are prevented by varied patterns of steps. Thus there is reduced risk of injury, which could otherwise occur by overtaxing individual sections of muscles or joints.

- Motivation:

  Music and the trainer's personality are important factors which motivate people to take part in aerobics classes regularly. Compared with endurance sports, which one does alone, aerobics courses give an opportunity for the participants to be motivated to train regularly and so benefit from the health-promoting effects of regular endurance training.

9.1 The Aerobics Trainer's Example

The factors mentioned under the heading "motivation", show that the personal charisma of the aerobics trainer plays a significant role. We are here talking about punctuality, professionalism in appearance and communicative abilities.

- Punctuality

   Give yourself enough time (at least 30 minutes) before your lesson starts, in order to concentrate on the following 60 minutes. Each lesson of the course is a fresh challenge which you should be prepared for. As trainer, you need time to switch off from the everyday world, run through the choreography in your mind, repeat the steps which are supposed to round off your choreography, think about your participants etc. Also, leave yourself enough time to wind back your music cassettes. Trainers who rush into the beginning of the lesson, transfer a sense of time pressure onto their participants leads in most cases to a hectic and badly-taught lesson.

- Professionalism in appearance

   Shoes and clothing should be of the same standard, which you expect from your participants. Many participants take their lead either consciously or sub-consciously from the trainer's external details. So you should wear shoes which do justice to the highest functional demands of a good aerobics shoe (stable, with cushioning features in the front and heel area). Clothing should be light and right for the time of year and the room temperature. Materials which have proved suitable are those which transfer any sweatiness back into the environment e.g. cotton-mixture fibres. Very loose clothing often hides the movement or body position which you wish to demonstrate to your participants, and makes teaching more difficult; on the other hand, close-fitting clothing should be discreet.

- Communicative abilities

   One of the most important deciding factors, whether the participants actually enjoy their aerobics classes and want to come again, is a positive atmosphere. Try and use positive statements like "you did that well!",

"I'm sure you are noticing that the knees are slightly bent" in preference to negative statements e.g. "That's wrong!", "Do not stretch the knees out!". If you employ this sort of strategy you will prove the well-tested theory that human-beings learn best with praise rather than with blame. Plan some time before and after your aerobics class for questions, observations or problems.

9.2 Extrinsic versus Intrinsic Motivation: Why One Trains

The success of each aerobics programme usually depends on how often it is done. How often it is run again is dependent on whether the participants enjoy physical activity i.e. depends on the participants' motivation.

Completely untrained people often feel physically uncomfortable at the start of a movement programme, and overstretched (muscle cramps, exhaustion). The desire to stop can last up to ten weeks with beginners who are training regularly. It is mainly external motives which help the participants not to give up, despite negative experience. Thoughts like "That is doing my health good" or "I'll get a better figure", are examples of such motives (extrinsic motivation – see box 1). A stage can be added to this exertion phase, where exertion and demanding too much can be eradicated by feelings of physical well-being, at least to conclude the sporting activity. The motivation can at this stage change into the direction of a larger number of intrinsic motives, characterised by feelings of happiness, relaxation and pleasure because of the physical activity itself.

The results of many investigations prove that intrinsic motivation is more likely to change one's attitude in the long term towards including sporting activities in one's daily round of activities. Of course it is extrinsic motives which cause most people to start some kind of sporting activity: either because they want greater performance potential in physical activity, want to control their weight or lose weight, or because they want to reduce their risk of illness; all these are valid reasons as the outcome of sporting activity. Although these extrinsic motives play a big role in determining whether anyone starts doing sport at all, there is the contradiction that permanent concentration on the expected results of sporting activity can impede the development of intrinsic motives and make it less likely that

Types of Motivation

EXTRINSIC MOTIVATION ("PRODUCT-ORIENTATED")	INTRINSIC MOTIVATION ("PROCESS-ORIENTATED")
Reduced risk of illness	"I feel good, when I do sport"
Weight control	Sport is fun
Future	Present
"I must"	"I want to"

physical activity becomes a habit in the long term. An important step from a position of extrinsic to intrinsic motivation lies in concentrating on the physical activity itself and on awareness of the feelings connected with this activity. When the sport being done corresponds to one's individual capabilities and needs, then the sportively active participants sense a high degree of satisfaction, self-control and happiness. This state is described in the English language as "flow", and is regarded as a central factor of intrinsic motivation.

To ease the changeover from extrinsic to intrinsic motivation, it has proved helpful to explain the participant's motivation in an interview. Such a conversation should help the participant to recognise his goals better, when doing sport. In the following interview there are some examples of questions which can be used as conversational guidelines:

Motivation Interview

MOTIVATING FACTOR	QUESTION
1. Personal goals	What would you like to achieve and why?
2. Personal willingness	What are you prepared to do?
3. Potential obstructions	What could prevent your reaching your goal?
4. Self-confidence	How confident are you that you can overcome the obstacles, we have just talked about?
5. Perceived advantages	What positive effects do you expect when you have reached your goal?

6. Figure problems	Do you not like others making remarks about your figure when you introduce yourself? Could this deter your taking part in group activity? If so how could we alter this? What could you do?
7. Social support	Do you need support or encouragement from others? If so, how do you get it?
8. Feelings	How do you feel when doing sport? How could you compare these feelings with other activities?
9. Happiness	What can you do to always make sport good fun? What can you do to get more enjoyment out of training?

Here are a few more motivating techniques to help participants be better-motivated to maintaining their aerobics programme.

Encouragement
Encourage your participants and praise their performance as this is probably the best way to strengthen their self-confidence. As aerobics trainer, you possess both the specialist and personal authority which makes your praise particularly valueable to your participants.

Set short-term goals
Conceptions within a training programme of what sort of goals should be attained and within what time limits, often have unrealistic ideals. One is more likely to succeed, when one takes small but continous steps towards the desired goal (e.g. losing weight) than if one puts a vast amount of effort into it. Suggest quickly-attainable and less-demanding goals to your participants.

Variability
By changing the floorwork exercises frequently, or with lots of different step sequences in the cardio-phase, you can make an aerobics class more interesting and avoid rapid tiredness and injuries caused by overtaxing certain muscles and joints.

Feeling of participation
Give your participants the feeling that you are happy to be with them, and if someone is missing, enquire about her, but without any kind of social pressure.

9.3 Dependence on Sport and Eating Disorders

More and more results of surveys point to the fact that there are people who feel compelled to carry out their training programme. The desire to train is sometimes so great that the body is permanently overstretched resulting in sport injuries. These sort of people react to interruptions in training with increased irrascibility and a general feeling of discomfort. They reduce all social contacts, so that they always have time for a steadily increasing amount of training. Finally, the training dominates other areas of their lives. Put all these aspects together and scientists talk about so-called dependence on sport, but they differentiate between two types: primary and secondary sport dependence. Primary sport dependence happens when sport is done in the way described above, without any other obvious psychological problem. On the other hand, one talks about secondary sport dependence, when the sport-dependent behaviour results from another psychological disorder and this is usually an eating disorder.

Eating Disorders

Daily contact with food is becoming a problem for more and more people. Whilst for one food becomes a tortuous obsession, for another fasting becomes an apparently incontrollable necessity. It is still mainly young women (teenagers and young adults) who are affected by unhealthy changes in their dietary behaviour, but the number of men is also increasing. The obsession of eating and then being sick (Bulimia Nervosa) is particularly widespread. Lasting for years, eating orgies occur, which are beyond the control of the affected people, so that they eat vast amounts of food in the shortest possible time and are then sick. Lots of Bulimia patients employ extreme methods to lose weight which end in a fatal circle. The affected person tries to reduce their often only assumed overweight by radical dieting and/or an excessive amount of sports training. This leads to exaggerated deficiencies, which the body tries to compensate at all costs. The desire to eat greedily becomes so overwhelming, that it can no longer be controlled. An eating orgy takes place, whereby, in a few hours, one catches up on all the eating which has been denied the body for days or even weeks. From the deep-rooted fear of putting on weight after such an attack, one is voluntarily sick and the diet is resumed more intensely, as well as more training being done. This results in the next eating-and-being-sick attack being preprogrammed; thus the fatal circle of fasting, excessive training, eating-and-being-sick attack, renewed fasting and training is complete.

The reason that it is mainly women who are affected by such eating disorders often comes from the desperate attempt to fit into society's ideal slim-figure concept. These women are often so much slaves to this pressure, that they frequently have quite the wrong outlook on their own body. The impression that they are too fat is not so much determined by looking in the mirror, as from a much-distorted and subjective view of their own body. The affected people feel unattractive and withdraw more and more. Their thinking goes round in circles with eating in the centre, together with the next diet and their figure. Such thought patterns are often expressed in restricted eating behaviour. Many of those affected say that they are always thinking about the calorie-content whilst eating. When and how much they eat bears no relation to the feelings of hunger or satisfying the body, but rather comes from irrational ideas about calories, putting on weight etc.

During an investigation at Marburg University, we examined the question how often such restricted eating behaviour can be found amongst leisure sportsmen. As well as asking about eating habits, we also looked into frequency of training and behaviour when injured by sport. The results indicate that about 10% of those questioned had a combination of restricted eating behaviour linked to their training behaviour, which come close to our suspecting possible sport dependence.

Naturally, the results of these surveys are not dependent on the place where the study was carried out or the people questioned. Surveys around other studios, sports and gymnastics clubs would probably reach different conclusions. In spite of this, or probably precisely because of it, such studies are necessary in order for us to identify trends in training and health behaviour of the people we aerobics trainers take care of, so that we can help individual cases. Unfortunately, we cannot ignore the fact that, in the future, with more and more people taking part in sport, the positive effects of sport are pushed aside or overrun by the negative effects of excessive training. The factors contributing to this development are many and various: they can be of a social, psychological or physiological nature (slimness-ideal, individual vulnerabilities or concepts about one's body). As aerobics trainers, we should make our course participants aware of the negative effects of too frequent and intensive training if we suspect that they have a problem.

10 The Health-political Meaning of Aerobics: Tasks and Opportunities

Although more people do sport today than several years ago, most children, young people and adults do not train enough, to derive the right illness-preventative benefits from physical activity. So we see it as one of our most important tasks to contribute to the future growth in sportively-active people in our society. The intrinsic fascination of aerobics could be a significant factor in our realising this aim.

When looking at the basic skills necessary for successful teaching, as discussed in this book, one requires correct step-technique and body posture, choreographic working with music, and a choice of safe and efficient exercises for the participants in line with recognised sports science ideals. These basic skills need continual practice and improvement. Knowledge already acquired about sports science's principles should be regularly revised and updated because of the rapid advance in health and sports scientific research.

As well as these basic skills, a good aerobics trainer is recognised by her being a sociable contact person and adviser about a healthy life-style. She should be able to give tips and information about healthy eating, advice about the correct amount of sporting activity, and finally be able to encourage periods of rest and relaxation. A prerequisite for such involvement is a lively interest in the needs and problems of the participants.

Aerobics trainers today are more than just good step-experts or choreographers. In the same way that the content and concept of aerobics sport has changed over the past two decades, so also has the desired profile of qualified aerobics teachers changed. It is a thing of the past that one could simply borrow a few exercises from other sports and put them to music. Today one needs a wide spectrum of knowledge, abilities and talents to teach an aerobics class well.

Yet in the middle of all these demands, "nobody is perfect". Rarely do we reach a permanent degree of perfection which is in line with the latest scientific research or the latest fashion. The quality of the trainer is not so much determined by an unrealistic level of perfectionism, as by her constant attempts to optimise her abilities and knowledge, and impart a sense of joy in living to her participants, which this wonderful kind of sport radiates.

Index

Literature

AMERICAN COUNCIL ON EXERCISE: Aerobics Instructor Manuel, San Diego 1993
(P.O. Box 910449, San Diego, CA 92191-0449 USA)

FREIWALD, J.: Aufwärmen im Sport – Übungen für Vorbereitung und Cool-Down, Rowohlt Hamburg 1991

KNEBEL, K.P.: Funktionsgymnastik, Rowohlt Hamburg 1987

KONOPKA, K.P.: Sporternährung, BLV Sportwissen 1988

VAITL, D. U. PETERMANN, F.: Handbuch der Entspannungsverfahren, Beltz PVU Weinheim 1993

WEINECK, J.: Optimales Training, Peri Med. Erlangen, 8. Auflage 1994

WEINECK, J.: Sportbiologie, Peri Med. Erlangen, 3. Auflage 1990

WIRHED, R.: Sport-Anatomie und Bewegungslehre, Schattauer, 2. Auflage 1988